7 Reasons to Believe in the Afterlife

"Dr. Charbonier teaches us that the brain is the link between the soul and the physical body and that it represents a set of structures optimized to create, record, and/or change patterns. When your brain dies your consciousness continues. Death is a transition to another life not an end in itself. When you are 'supposedly' dead; you are more alive than before!"

THE REV. KAREN E. HERRICK, PH.D., PRESIDENT OF THE ACADEMY OF SPIRITUALITY AND CONSCIOUSNESS STUDIES AND AUTHOR OF *YOU'RE NOT FINISHED YET*

"It is very refreshing to see such an important subject as NDEs and end-of-life experiences being taken seriously by a very experienced intensive care doctor. This is an interesting book that highlights the need to acknowledge and incorporate spiritual aspects of life into patient care as well as the need for a new understanding of consciousness."

PENNY SARTORI, PH.D., AUTHOR OF *THE WISDOM OF NEAR- DEATH EXPERIENCES*

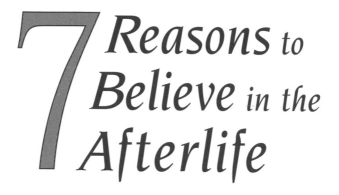

7 Reasons to Believe in the Afterlife

A DOCTOR REVIEWS THE CASE FOR CONSCIOUSNESS AFTER DEATH

JEAN JACQUES CHARBONIER, M.D.

TRANSLATED BY JACK CAIN

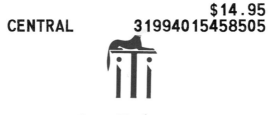

Inner Traditions
Rochester, Vermont • Toronto, Canada

Inner Traditions
One Park Street
Rochester, Vermont 05767
www.InnerTraditions.com

Library of Congress Cataloging-in-Publication Data
Charbonier, Jean Jacques.
  [7 bonnes raisons de croire à l'au-delà. English]
  7 reasons to believe in the afterlife : a doctor reviews the case for consciousness after death / Jean Jacques Charbonier, M.D. — First U.S. edition.
       pages cm
  Includes bibliographical references and index.
  ISBN 978-1-62055-380-0 (pbk.) — ISBN 978-1-62055-381-7 (e-book)
  1. Future life. 2. Near-death experiences. 3. Spiritualism. I. Title. II. Title: Seven reasons to believe in the afterlife.
  BL535.C514413 2015
  129—dc23
                                                                    2014038337

Printed and bound in the United States by Versa Press, Inc.
10 9 8 7 6 5 4 3 2 1

Text design and layout by Virginia Scott Bowman
This book was typeset in Garamond Premier Pro, Gill Sans, and Legacy Sans with Helvetica Neue and Novarese used as display typefaces

Contents

Acknowledgments

Many thanks to my wife, Corinne, who had the patience to accept all those moments taken up by my work as an intensive-care physician and also by my time-consuming activity as a writer and lecturer.

"He who is right twenty-four hours before the others is considered crazy for twenty-four hours only." Today we have arrived at the twenty-third hour and with all my heart I thank the scientists who dared to compromise their reputations by supporting my ideas. Dr. Olivier Chambon and Emmanuel Ransford had that courage. For that, I offer them my infinite gratitude.

As well, I would like to thank all of the "Leos" who inspired the drafting of this book. Without them, it would not have come to be. I would also like to thank all of the "Gabriels" (who most often were—as was I at the time I was finishing my studies in medicine—repentant former "Leos").

Foreword

Take note: This book is a public utility venture! In ten or fifteen years what Dr. Charbonier is affirming today, namely the survival of consciousness after death, will probably seem like the most ordinary thing in the world. But today he is alone in having the courage to affirm this with great clarity, using science as his foundation. And this he has done in spite of virulent and sometimes personal attacks directed at him from materialists and skeptics of all persuasions.

Writing in a lively, easy to read style, and taking into account the latest scientific discoveries, J. J. Charbonier shows us just how important it is to reconsider our point of view about death. In this study, you will learn that the best reason for believing in the hereafter arises from the fact that the hypothesis of life after death is now much more valid than the opposite materialist view that affirms that after death there is nothing. The good doctor bases his position on data collected from numerous scientific studies carried out over the last thirty-five years.

Just the case of Pamela Reynolds alone (as recounted in the next chapter), and the way in which Jean Jacques Charbonier refutes the unfounded materialist objections to it, demonstrates his position. Her case proves all by itself that consciousness is independent of the brain and survives the death of the brain. Dr. Charbonier's book might well have borrowed its title—*The End of Materialism*—from a book by the scientist Charles Tart. One need only look at the facts that have been brought to light: Doubt is no longer in the picture and materialism has lost the debate.

There is very definitely a life of consciousness that continues after the death of the body. My colleague suggests that the expression "experience of provisional death" would be an improvement over "near-death experience" (NDE). As he puts it so well,

> Someone whose heart stops is not "near death," or "on the borders of death," or "in a state of imminent death"—he is *already* dead and may have been dead for quite a few minutes. Some people claim, erroneously in my view, that NDE "is like being in the departure lounge of an airport—you haven't really gotten on the plane and you don't really know the destination." Rather than that, during an NDE everything seems to indicate that we *do* take the plane, that we really do arrive in the land of the dead, but we come back, because we were lucky enough to have a return ticket, unlike the usual irreversible death.

In this practical manual, we really are talking about death and what happens after life on Earth. What you have in your hands is something like a "road map for the afterlife," a way of preparing yourself for your own passing, or helping to prepare those close to you for theirs, so that the person concerned is in a position to take advantage of this "final journey."

Individuals who have lived through this contact with death are quick to say that what happened to them is "more real than reality" and that any doubts about the existence of the hereafter is, for them, pointless. They no longer fear death, and their spiritual transformation in the years following their experience is in itself a major argument supporting the authenticity of their contact with another reality. As Professor Kenneth Ring has shown, the long-term, very positive impact of an NDE on the existence of those who have been through one can be partially transmitted, like a sort of positive virus, to those who read the accounts of these "experiencers."

In the study that you now have in your hands I believe you will catch this virus and it will change your life! In the long term, it brings laughter, love, and joy to everyday life. And in facing life, it is easier to relax when you know that it will continue after the death of the body. Only that which is essential—our consciousness, our knowledge, our capacity to love, and our loving connections—is carried over into the hereafter.

I will conclude this foreword by giving you my heartfelt response, which arose just after I finished reading this book and which I immediately expressed in a note to Dr. Charbonier:

> Dear colleague, I have just finished reading your book: how lively, clear, and convincing it is! I am sure it will become a reference work that will open minds and touch hearts in the public at large. With what clarity you set forth the facts as well as all those beautiful firsthand accounts. And with what skill you unravel the arguments of your (our) materialist detractors, so predictable in their naïve unseeingness. Bravo and thank you for all of this. Death's lessons teach us how to live better!
>
> Olivier Chambon, M.D.

Olivier Chambon has been a psychiatrist and psychotherapist for more than twenty years and is a pioneer of behavioral and cognitive methods of care for chronically psychotic patients. In France, he is responsible for co-creating the university degree known as integrative psychotherapy. Trained in shamanism and in many disciplines of psychotherapy, he is the author of *La medicine psychédélique* (Psychedelic Medicine) and the coauthor, with Laurent Huguelit, of *Le chamane et le psy* (The Shaman and the Shrink).

Preface

People often ask me, "Doctor, you said that you are convinced of the existence of the hereafter. Do you have at least one good reason you can give to back that up?" Or: "I know you have written several books on life after this life. I'm looking for a book that isn't full of medical terminology and is not too hard to read and which I can give to someone who is very open to all these things but hasn't read anything about them. What title would you advise?"

These frequently asked questions led me to write this book. I was looking for a text that would be as simple and concise as possible. I wanted it to provide answers—for an uninitiated readership—to classic questions from a novice and to be a book that could also answer questions from most of the skeptics and materialist detractors who consistently assail me through the Internet and the media.

I have sought out the best arguments to support the existence of a hereafter and I have found seven of them—seven phenomena that are unfortunately quite unknown, disputed by many people, and yet irrefutable—seven stunning proofs that are difficult to counter. For each one of them I have provided space for their detractors to speak so that I may expose the weakness of their reasoning and show that such reasoning easily crumbles in the face of the logic of a rigorous and objective analysis. Belief in a hereafter transforms life. Material values fade and are no longer a priority; fear of death disappears; happiness becomes synonymous with love and spirituality and, because of this, it seems much more accessible.

In this lower world dominated by money, however, we are egoistically driven to desire to accumulate material riches while disregarding everything else. And certainly it is because of this that there are so many unhappy people in our Western society. We no longer talk to each other in depth and meditation is considered a waste of time! It seems indeed to be atypical, in this materialistic culture, to value giving love to others by taking full advantage of the fortuitous instances of a random encounter, or at any particular moment indulge in a walk in nature, or seize an opportunity to have a prolonged conversation with a friend or a stranger whom we happen to run into by chance.

A belief in the hereafter is capable of shifting this paradigm for, as we shall see, a transcendent modification related to a belief in the hereafter takes place in 18 percent of the people who have a heart attack and in all people who have a sincere, real faith in God. Belief in a hereafter also has the advantage of improving health. In fact, the positive effect of faith and prayer on sickness has attracted the attention of numerous physicians. A survey published in the November 10, 2003, issue of *Newsweek* revealed that a faith in God strengthens morale and promotes an easier and quicker return to good health after a serious illness. In the same study, it was found that 72 percent of Americans think that prayer helps one to heal better by fostering an early recovery. Work conducted at Rush University in Chicago, as well as research at the University of Michigan, showed that depression and psychosomatic illness linked to stress occurred less frequently in believers, and the mortality rate of young adults was reduced by 25 percent in those who believed in life after death. Duke University in North Carolina determined that this same rate decreased 30 percent in heart patients in the year after a serious operation if these patients practiced prayer.

These scientific studies only confirm what many of us have believed for years: Belief in the existence of a hereafter provides a greater resiliency and buoyancy in the face of life's challenges and, at the same time, diminishes the serious physical repercussions connected with stress, anxiety, and fear. I invite you now to travel with me on this journey to the other side. It may change the way you view all that you have come to know thus far.

Note to the Reader

The accounts contained in this book are authentic; they have been personally addressed to me in writing or confided to me in interviews. At the request of certain individuals, however, I have sometimes used fictitious identities and removed any material that might identify the persons concerned. In providing these accounts, I had to limit myself to extracts from the correspondence I received.

If, after finishing this book, you liked it, please don't shelve it in your library where it will sleep. Instead, give it away! Among your acquaintances—relatives, friends, and, why not? even your enemies—choose the one person who seems the most skeptical about the existence of the hereafter and give it to him or her as a gift. Write a sentence or two on the first page as a dedication, with a date and your signature below it. Then, just wait. . . . If you have any news from your unlikely reader in the following days, weeks, or months, please write to me. I collect all sorts of reactions to add to my personal statistics and in preparation for my next book.

May this plea in favor of a hereafter open doors toward real serenity and better health, in spite of the sometimes cruel and painful moments of life.

The 1st Good Reason

Sixty Million People Who Came Back from the Dead

And if you are convinced that something doesn't exist, you don't see it.

ERVIN LASZLO, INREES (*INSTITUT DE RECHERCHE SUR LES EXPÉRIENCES EXTRAORDINAIRES* [RESEARCH INSTITUTE FOR EXTRAORDINARY EXPERIENCES]), PARIS, MAY 25, 2011

Right after my heart stopped beating, I left my body. I was at the ceiling and I saw everything—I watched all the details of my resuscitation. I wanted to shout at the people who were trying to bring me back to life to leave me alone, to let me leave, but they couldn't hear me. I felt really great and didn't have the slightest desire to return to my body. Then I moved into a tunnel. I was bathed in a light of unconditional love and my happiness was indescribably powerful. I saw once again my whole life in great detail and in fast-forward. I felt the good and the bad that I had done to others.

I met a light being of infinite goodness who asked me what I had made of my life and what I had done for others. My deceased parents came to welcome me and to say that I had to go back to my body because unfortunately I could not stay with them no matter how badly I wanted to. They showed me a boundary, which was a limit that I was not to cross. At the moment that I came back into my body, all my earthly pain came back and I was terribly sad to leave this marvelous light.

I am now very happy because I know that there is life after death and that one day I will be once again in this light of love. I also know that, on this Earth, the most important thing is to know how to love and help others. This experience has turned my life upside down. Nothing will ever be the same as before.

JOURNEYS
TOWARD THE HEREAFTER

During twenty-five years of practicing intensive care medicine, I have been able to gather several hundred accounts of patients who returned from clinical death. The text of the story above has been pieced together by condensing and synthesizing these accounts; it is a kind of summary that brings together the main elements of these remarkable journeys to the hereafter. The event sequence described is almost always the same, and this is true regardless of culture, philosophy, geographic location, and religion.

There is no one factor that determines who will undergo this experience. Age, sex, social standing, belief system—none of these bear on the specific predisposition to undergo this extraordinary experience. At the same time, each story is unlike any other story because each person has their own expression of the experience, with their own sensitivity and culture. Nevertheless, numerous elements recur in the stories I was able to collect, leading one to imagine that, with very few exceptions, the route is always the same.

It's as if a young Inuit, an elderly American woman, and a gentleman from Senegal in his fifties each went on a trip to Venice, Italy, and then relayed their accounts. Their stories would be very different, but, all in all, we would be able to make out rather quickly that the three persons had visited the same city. For example, a child who had suffered cardiac arrest said, in describing a being of light, that he had seen "a tall man who was lighting himself up all on his own." Some people meet Jesus Christ, others Buddha, the Virgin Mary, or the Prophet Muhammad. The divine personage seen in the light changes according to one's belief system and religion.

One element is found consistently in one hundred percent of the cases: For those who have had this experience, they know that life continues after death and the hereafter exists. They are intimately convinced of this and nothing or no one is able to change their minds. One such person said to me one day: "Even if a scientist manages to prove through logic that my experience was only a hallucination, I would not believe him for an instant because I am certain deep down that what I experienced that day was totally real—it had nothing to do with a dream or a hallucination!"

According to the latest statistical studies, there are at least 60 million people who have had this transcendental experience following cardiac arrest: 4 percent of the population of the West (12 million Americans, 2.5 million French). There are fewer cases in areas of the world where facilities for resuscitation don't really exist.[1] It's very likely, however, that, as these accounts become better known, we will very quickly see an increase of them.

It must also be said that, in a small number of cases, ventures into the hereafter are experienced in a way that isn't all that pleasant or marvelous. Michel Garant, for example, still has a terrible memory of his experience under anesthesia during his coronary bypass operation, which was conducted in near-emergency conditions in 1997. His story shows clearly all the negative sides of his experience. Several studies have been carried out to try and understand why certain individuals have a brush with hell instead of paradise and, in these cases as well, no predictive factor seems to emerge.

The following is Michel's account.

We never know how things will go as we pass to the other side of the mirror. The poet Verlaine wrote, "Often I dream a strange and piercing dream. . . . " The music of this poem and many others kept me company as I was wheeled to the operating room . . .

What was I going to dream?

The blinding spotlights, the arms crossed, the green angels that buzzed around the sacrificial altar . . .

Like the pelican in the poem, I was going to have my body torn apart right to the guts, right to the heart that had begun to beat too wildly!

A voice said, "Close your fist. I'm going to squeeze your arm then find your best vein. You won't feel a thing. Then start counting."

A slight burning sensation ran through the vein in my left arm and I counted . . . "one, two, three, four, five," and then there was nothing but the soft, sweet, cottony descent toward the void. . . . Emptiness, absence, the undefined. I don't know how long I wandered without perception . . .

I awoke suddenly, tiny and naked, icy on the inside more than on the outside. I found myself stuck on an endless wall that had no base and no top, without beginning or end. All I could see was this grainy beige wall that some unknown force was pressing me against, crushing me into, laminating me onto. . . . I was afraid, I was alone, far from everything, far from everyone, far from sound, alone, a tiny naked baby in an icy silence. . . . I was cold, terribly cold. Then, terrified, I felt this horrible wall move, tilt, dragging me toward the void. . . . I was about to fall into absolute horror. . . . So, then that's what this is . . . DEATH . . . or HELL . . .

But no, I regained awareness of my icy body. I heard noise around me. Noise is so reassuring. . . . The voices of the angels who were saying, "He's waking up. . . ." I was cold—so cold. I wanted someone to cover me with a warm blanket but I was encased in ice, my body would not respond, it no longer obeyed my commands . . .

Why have I been locked in this inert body that is my prison?

I wanted to scratch the sheet that I was lying on but that too was impossible—my hands were frozen stiff.

Finally I was able to say, "I'm cold . . ."

Another example: This extract from an account by C. L.—who for obvious reasons of confidentiality wanted to remain anonymous—illustrates perfectly what can be a hellish experience during cardiac arrest.

I was at the ceiling and I was watching the anesthetist massaging my heart, doing CPR [cardiac pulmonary resuscitation] on me while the surgeon was asking him what he was supposed to do. It was easy to recognize my body on the operating table, but it was like someone else's body—one that already no longer belonged to me. There were a lot of people around me trying to revive me. Then I entered a kind of very dark cone that was turning in a spiral, and a strong current carried me toward the end of this funnel. As I was moving through, I passed grimacing, furrowed faces that seemed to belong to people who were in terrible suffering. The further I penetrated into this cylinder that was becoming narrower and narrower, the more deeply these people were suffering. They cried out but no sound came from their lips. It was awful. I was able to also feel their suffering in myself. [. . .]

When I finally arrived in front of an immense flame, I at first thought I was in hell and that I would burn up immediately. But the flame began to dance in a funny way and it wrapped itself around me, asking how I had helped others. I didn't know how to answer. At that moment I became aware that the life I had been leading was nothing but a string of petty thefts and pathetic swindlings. I had thought only of how to benefit myself by stealing from others and despising them. I was really miserable because I had helped no one, least of all myself. My near-death experience [NDE] showed me that only in helping others could one be happy. And that is what I do now.

My NDE also gave me the chance to be able to treat others using my hands. I did this spontaneously from the moment I was back in my life. I treat without charging and that's okay. My friends no longer recognize me because I used to be a businessman who thought only of the almighty dollar. Now I am completely without resources and, above all, completely free. I have no fear of death because I know that I will

have good deeds to show when I come in front of God once again. The
moral is that we can only be happy when we help others, even if it's just
helping someone cross the street.

Djoharsi Ahmed is a psychoanalyst with a doctorate in psychopa-
thology. Fascinated for a long time by altered states of consciousness
and telepathic phenomena, she is one of those rare scientists who has
integrated the spiritual dimension into her various therapies. We asked
her what she thought of these experiences of hell. Here is her reply.

A positive NDE is a remarkable state of turning narcissistically to one-
self, a fusion with absolute love, and an almost all-encompassing com-
prehension of oneself. The negative NDEs are the opposite, term for
term, of the positive NDEs: What was magnificent becomes diabolical,
what was beauty becomes horror and anguish, what was light becomes
darkness, and paradise becomes hell. The most difficult thing for some-
one who has had a negative NDE is to speak about it because there is
a lot of guilt running through it. "If others have such a beautiful experi-
ence and I have such a terrifying one, I must be a real monster!" That
is why it's important to tell people about the experience—it needs to be
integrated by the person who experienced it.

I have had numerous discussions with people who had dis-
agreeable experiences following cardiac arrest. They are much more

hesitant to provide their accounts than those who had marvelous feelings of indescribable happiness. It's true that it's not very encouraging or wonderful to claim that you've encountered hell! However, I've noticed that the vast majority of this group of "unfortunate ones" retain a rather positive memory of the adventure. They are no longer afraid of death—which might at first glance seem very paradoxical given what they encountered when everything fell apart. Instead, they have integrated their negative experience as a warning from the hereafter, which asks them to *change their behavior on this planet by giving love to others.*

These individuals are convinced that by modifying the whole gamut of their life's goals, they will be following a different path from the one they experienced at the moment of their provisional death. Some even say that they have once again found a faith in God that they had been missing for a very long time. In short, these negative experiences of provisional death were, in these cases, experienced as a good lesson being provided by the hereafter.

THE EXPERIENCE IS NOT A HALLUCINATION

Today the majority of scientists still assume that the transcendent experience must result from a hallucinatory phenomenon produced by a failing brain that has been deprived of oxygen and has a surfeit of carbon dioxide. These skeptics suggest that a deficit of oxygen in a poorly supplied occipital lobe of the brain can provoke visions of points of light that resemble the end of a tunnel and that metabolic disturbances provoked by a prolonged cerebral hypoxia (a lack of oxygen) will give rise to sensations of intense pleasure by activating morphine receptors. As for the sensation of leaving the body, (according to them) it can be induced by the stimulation of a precise area of the brain: the right angular gyrus. This is a coherent explanation—even though totally invented—which sees all the fleeting sensations perceived during an NDE integrated with multiple memories from one's life, and the whole being spontaneously reconstituted by the brain once it recovers its autonomy.

These explanations don't stand up to scrutiny for very long when you have a thorough familiarity with near-death experiences. Let's look at this rationale in more detail now.

OXYGEN DEFICIT AND SURPLUS OF CARBON DIOXIDE

We know that hypoxia (again, a lack of oxygen) and hypercapnia (an excess of carbon dioxide) produce fairly typical specific clinical indicators that include slow thinking, irritability, difficulty concentrating, and memory issues—in short, behavior that is in sharp contrast with the perception of mental clarity experienced by people undergoing an NDE.

Dr. Pim van Lommel is a cardiologist in Holland who has devoted a great deal of his time to the study of NDEs. He reported the very interesting case of a man whose levels of oxygen and carbon dioxide in the blood were measured following a cardiac arrest and at the precise moment of the NDE. Although the patient seemed completely unconscious, he clearly "saw" the doctor introduce a needle in his femoral artery in order to analyze the gases carried in the blood. The results of this examination were perfectly normal; there was no hypoxia or hypercapnia. The fact that this examination took place at the exact moment of the NDE—since the patient was at that moment outside his body observing what was transpiring—shows very clearly that NDEs are not the result of a lack of oxygen or an excess of carbon dioxide.

Regarding the enveloping light of love that is experienced by those undergoing an NDE, skeptics claim that the vision of a point of light induced by a poorly supplied occipital lobe creates an image that looks like an old television set with a cathode ray tube (CRT) screen that has just been turned off; the intensity of a luminous spot gets bigger quickly and then gradually decreases before disappearing completely. However, one need only interview those brought back from death to realize that the appearance of a CRT screen being turned off has absolutely nothing in common with the accounts of an indescribable light of love bursting forth at the end of a tunnel. That light is increasing in intensity and volume. It never looks like a luminous flash that fades little by little.

The following is Paul Brunet's account of what happened to him during a motorcycle accident.

At the end of this dark corridor that I was plunging through at incredible speed, there was a light that was more powerful than a trillion suns but was not blinding me. When I got close to it, it completely enveloped me; I was bathed in it. The light loved me. It spoke to me telepathically. Never in my life have I encountered anything so powerful and so loving as this divine light.

The stimulation of the morphine receptors of the brain can certainly give rise to a sensation of extraordinary well-being and produce the specific pleasure that morphine addicts seek. But to my knowledge, a hit of morphine, as powerful as it may be, has never been enough to change someone's life in as radical a way as the NDEs we are speaking about here do. Actually, after this out-of-the-ordinary adventure, we often see spectacular upsets: people divorce; move house; change jobs, friends, and/or subjects of interest, for instance. If the experience is totally integrated and accepted, relationships with others are improved as the personality becomes more loving and more attractive. Some people say they have gone on to develop artistic, intuitive, channeling, or healing faculties. These are not things you usually see in a morphine addict!

It is true that the stimulation of the right angular gyrus produces the impression of being slightly shifted out of the body—an "external autoscopy vision"—which can give the person the illusion of seeing their own body from outside of it.[2] However, this reproducible hallucinatory phenomenon can't be compared to what is undergone in the NDE, wherein certain subjects are capable of describing not only their body as if they were outside it or at some distance above it but also precise details that would be impossible to recount unless the viewer was some distance away. These precise details have included, for example, a plaque hidden below the operating table,[3] all the various movements made by the medical team during a cardiac arrest, the drawer where the denture of the patient being resuscitated was hastily put away,[4] the numbers on the license plate of a hit-and-run driver who left the pedestrian for dead (while the pedestrian had in fact "seen" the whole thing),[5] and many other elements of the same kind that are too tedious to list here, given that they are so numerous.

A coherent story made up by a failing brain cannot explain how subjects were able to describe precise situations taking place far from their bodies, such as an operation taking place in an adjoining hospital room, the apparel and postures of people in the waiting room,[6] the number of bicycles lined up in the hospital parking lot,[7] or a very specific scene that was taking place in an apartment located miles away. Everything takes place, in fact, as if the consciousness of the resuscitated subject was able to move through walls to witness precise events that, after detailed investigation, turn out to be real.

Here is Geneviève Rodriguez's account that illustrates this point.

While the firemen were performing CPR on me, I left my body through the top of my skull, moved through the walls of the operating room and the hospital, and finally arrived at the home of my parents, who were crying. My brother was also with them and it really surprised me to see him there because for a long time he had been angry with Mom and Dad and had refused to see them. The most amazing thing was that I later learned that my brother really was *with my parents at that moment.*

How could a failing brain make up a story when it didn't have most of the elements? In a case like this, where is the information located? The simplest explanation is certainly to assume that a separated consciousness existed during the experience. You will readily agree that there isn't any explanation that is more logical than this.

When I am interviewed about NDEs for televised documentaries or news reports, it always happens that, following what I have said, a colleague who is a psychiatrist, neurologist, or emergency-medicine physician contradicts my conclusions regarding the hypothesis of a separated consciousness while, at the same time, defending the theory of a hallucinating, dying brain. It's amusing to notice that the journalist will usually present this colleague who is arguing against me with a preemptory, "Now let's hear the opinion of a scientist!" even though said scientist has had the same university education that I've had and even though I've been interested in this subject for much longer than he has. It certainly would appear that, for the commentator in question, a physician engaged in resuscitation who suggests the existence of a separated consciousness cannot be a scientist!

MEETING DECEASED PEOPLE

It very often happens that during an NDE that subject meets relatives or friends who have passed. A most disturbing aspect of this is that, in certain cases, they don't know at the time of the experience that these acquaintances had already died! They receive confirmation of that only when they come back![8] It's obvious that this astonishing information cannot be produced by a hallucination.

More surprising still is the case of Mathieu Meilleur who, during his NDE, met a person whom he had absolutely never met before. Several days after his NDE, his girlfriend "happened" to show him a photo of her former boyfriend who had been killed in a motorcycle accident. Mathieu Meilleur immediately recognized the unfortunate motorcycle driver as being the same as the person whom he had met in his NDE!

BLIND PERSONS' NDES

Another argument to refute the hallucination theory: blind people are able to provide visual information about their resuscitations. Whether their handicap is congenital or acquired, they are able to see for the first time or see once again during their NDEs. Several researchers[9] have pored over this incomprehensible scenario without being able to provide any explanation for it.

How might it be possible to see without eyes?

THEY REALLY HAVE COME BACK
FROM THE DEAD!

Subjects who have lived through these experiences really have come back from the dead. Clinical death is defined as the cessation of brain function. This state can be determined by recording the absence of neuronal electrical activity—a flat electroencephalogram (EEG). When there have been two flat EEGs four hours apart for a duration of twenty minutes—except for conditions of narcosis (wherein intravenous products have been administered to produce sleep) or hypothermia—we consider that clinical death has become irreversible. In such conditions we are free to disconnect the patient from a respirator or to remove organs for donation. In fact, this state corresponds to our current limits of resuscitation and probably a few decades from now we will have gone well beyond these limits. We need to remember that doctors in former generations did not do CPR and were comfortable with signing a death certificate as soon as a heart stopped beating.

Recently we have become aware that an EEG flatlines within fifteen seconds of a cardiac arrest. Given that, under the best surveillance conditions—which is the case in intensive care units—there is a minimum period of at least a minute before initial procedures can be brought to bear. Given this, we can be assured that all victims resuscitated following cardiac arrest have certainly undergone clinical death. (There are people in the country whose hearts began beating again after several tens of minutes, subsequent to intervention by the closest emergency medicine unit!)

Our studies have shown that about 18 percent[10] of the subjects resuscitated from a cardiac arrest relate the amazing experience described at the beginning of this chapter. The term "near-death experience" used in the English-speaking world since the 1970s and the terms used in French, *"experience de mort imminente"* (EMI)—the experience of imminent death—or *"experience aux frontiers de la mort"* (EFM)—an experience at the borders of death—are now completely outmoded terms. It is now more appropriate to speak of an "experience of provisional death" (EPD). Clinical death is, in fact, already present when patients are resuscitated because brain activity is absent from the moment the first CPR action begins. A person whose heart has stopped is not "near death," nor "on the borders of death," nor "in a state of imminent death." He or she is *already* dead and often has been dead for quite a few minutes!

I know by heart the speech that my detractors make: "These people were not dead because they came back!" Or I hear: "Just because there is no detectable electrical activity does not mean that the brain is no longer functioning. Perhaps there is a residual activity that we are as yet unable to measure!"

On the first point, the answer is easy. The definition of clinical death is unequivocal and we have objective proof: When a heart has stopped, in less than a minute a cessation of all detectable cerebral activity follows. Subjects have returned from these states of clinical death because emergency medical teams set off to get them back. If no one had resuscitated them, they would never have come back! Like it or not, they have certainly known death and 18 percent of them tell us about a journey that is almost identical in all respects.

As for undetectable residual cerebral activity, even if we accept this difficult to refute argument, it nevertheless remains faulty. It provides absolutely no explanation for how, in a period of cardiac arrest, a brain would be capable of producing a state of consciousness that is working better than when it's in an ordinary situation of proper functioning—never mind allowing for what appears to be the ability of consciousness to move about in time and space, to pass through walls, and to communicate via telepathy, among other extraordinary feats and conditions.

Sixty million people who have returned from the dead have the potential to describe the hereafter to us. Among all these fantastic stories, we will necessarily find the tales of lunatics or charlatans who are trying to get on the bandwagon. It's up to us to identify them with a maximum of vigilance, care, and discernment. Since the scientific proof of a life after this life is based solely on eyewitness accounts, the greatest difficulty will be to find the tools to unmask the imposters.

Most doctors think that the brain is a kind of gland that secretes consciousness just as the pancreas produces insulin. This belief is so strong that it is totally impossible for them to imagine that at the moment when this organ stops working, consciousness could still exist. The unique and incontrovertible case reported in the next chapter formally demonstrates the opposite. This unusual case, observed during a brain operation, revolutionizes all of our paradigms about death. On December 15, 2001, this topic was the subject of a paper in the very serious academic journal *The Lancet*.[11] There is nothing esoteric about this journal and yet the article in question, written by cardiologist Pim van Lommel, proves that a consciousness—and therefore life—is still capable of existing following the confirmed death of the brain. This case alone plunges us into a well of reflection about what might happen to us at the moment of our *own* death.

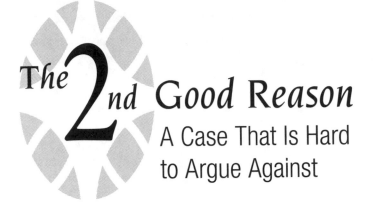

The 2nd Good Reason
A Case That Is Hard to Argue Against

Such are men with little learning that the weakness of their minds prevents them from embracing and understanding the universal adaptability and harmony of all things.

SAINT AUGUSTINE, THE ORDER, I, 2

TWICE DEAD

Pamela Reynolds died on May 29, 2010, at the age of fifty-three, nineteen years after experiencing an earlier clinical death that had been medically induced by a surgical team whose goal was to remove a large aneurism lodged in her brainstem. Prior to the initial procedure, Dr. Robert Spetzier had hesitated a long time before undertaking the "last chance" operation. The risks were enormous, and yet if he didn't proceed with the intervention, the young woman was likely to suffer a premature demise. Her vascular tumor, lodged at the base of the brain, was like a veritable time bomb that, as it enlarged, could explode at any moment. Did they really have a choice?

It's worth going into some detail about the preparations for Pam's operation because it illustrates the extent to which her brain was inactive at the moment the vascular malformation was being removed. The "hypothermic circulatory arrest" (also called a *standstill operation*) that she benefited from is a technique used in extremely serious cases and only rarely because many patients are unable to withstand the disruption of blood flow that such an operation engenders. As a result, they die before the intervention can be successfully completed. This procedure involves the diversion of all blood flow from the area of the operation—the brain in Pam's case—to a circulatory system outside of her body. When underway, the individual must be in a state of hypothermia in order that the formation of irreversible brain lesions—which ordinarily takes place within five minutes of the cessation of cerebral blood flow—does not occur.

Having anesthetized Pam with a strong dose of barbiturates, the team diverted her blood flow outside her body while progressively lowering her temperature to the record level of 15.5°C (59.9°F). Then the surgical table on which the patient was lying was tilted steeply to ensure that Pam's brain would no longer contain a single drop of blood. As you might expect, the EEG quickly flatlined and stayed that way for almost an hour.

The intervention took place without any major problems. Once the aneurism was removed, there was nothing more to do but to await the patient's awakening to determine her neurological state. The first surprise was that Pam had suffered virtually no aftereffects from this artificially induced cerebral death. The second surprise was even more stunning: Her state of confirmed clinical death—

controlled and incontrovertible—in no way had prevented her from observing everything that had taken place around her during the operation! Yes, with a brain completely off-line, she was able to see, hear, and understand the smallest details of her surgery! This is a simply impossible feat if we believe that consciousness is fabricated by the brain.

Her astounding account is capable of causing any scientific materialist to jump up and down in indignation! Here is Pam's story.

I heard a mechanical noise and it reminded me of a dentist's drill. Then, I just sort of popped out of the top of my head. In this state, I was able to see the situation very clearly. I remember that my doctor had an instrument in his hand that looked like the handle of my electric toothbrush. It had a dent in it—a groove at the top where the tip appeared to go into the handle, but when I saw it, there was no tip. I looked down and saw a box; it reminded me of my father's box of tools when I was a child. That's where he kept his pocket wrenches.

At about the same moment that I saw the instrument, I heard a woman's voice. I believe it was the voice of my cardiologist. She was saying that my veins and arteries were too small to extract blood from them and the surgeon told her to try the other side. Feeling a presence, I sort of turned around to look at it, and it was then that I saw the tiny pinpoint of light. It seemed very far away and when I came closer to it, I heard my grandmother call me. I went to her right away and she kept me close.

The more I approached the light, the more I began to see people I recognized. I was impressed by the fact that these people had a marvelous look about them. My grandmother didn't look like an old woman;

she was radiant. Everyone looked young, healthy, and strong. I can say that they were of the light, as if they were wearing clothing made of light and as if they themselves were made of light. I was not allowed to go very far—they were keeping me close to them. I wanted to know more about the music, about the sound of a waterfall, about the birdsongs I was hearing, and I wanted to know why they wouldn't let me go farther.

They communicated with me. I have no other way of explaining it because they weren't speaking to me—they weren't speaking as you and I do. They thought—and I understood. They didn't want me to go into the light. They said that if I went too far, they would no longer be able to reconnect me to my physical self. My uncle led me down through the tunnel, and during the whole journey I really wanted to return to my body. I had no problem with that. I wanted to go back to my family.

Then I arrived near my body. I looked at it and frankly—it looked like a train wreck. It looked like what it was: dead, and I didn't want to go back into it any more. My uncle told me that it was like jumping into a swimming pool: "Go ahead, jump into the pool!" I was still holding back. And then something happened that I still don't understand even now—he sped up my return to the body by giving me a push just like when someone pushes you into a pool. When I touched my body it was as if I had fallen into a basin of icy water—and that I will never forget.

Beyond Pam's moving description of the hereafter, the precision she provides about the details of her operation supply all the ingredients for the greatest of scientific enigmas. What is there after death? What do we become? Where do we go? Where do we come from? These are the eternal, fundamental questions that flood into our minds starting at about the age of seven and which we then try to forget using all kinds of "distractions," none of which really work.

While in a deep coma Pamela Reynolds was able to describe the surgical instrument that was used to operate on her. She was also able to describe the metal box of instruments that indeed looked like a toolbox but the depth of which prevented one from seeing into its contents unless one was well above the level at which the operation was taking place. Moreover, Pam was able to accurately report the conversation between the cardiologist and the surgeon when her blood vessels were too flat to introduce suction tubes into them. All of this she did while her brain was no longer functioning. That means that this patient saw without her eyes, heard without her ears, and understood without her brain!

Yes, but with *what*?

How?

Again, doesn't the whole thing become a lot simpler if we accept that consciousness is found outside the body when the brain stops functioning?

WHAT THE DETRACTORS SAY

Pamela's EEG was flat but that doesn't mean there wasn't an unmeasurable residual activity.

False, because you must remember that the patient's body temperature had been lowered to 15.5°C (59.9°F) and we know that in such a condition there's no chance of having even the slightest biochemical exchange between two neurons. All brain functions are therefore out of the question.

Pamela's sensation of leaving the body arose from a stimulation of the right temporal lobe induced by a lack of oxygen

in relation to the lowering of blood pressure in the cerebral arteries and caused by the anesthetic, the hypothermia, and the draining of blood from the brain.

False, because a stimulation of the right temporal lobe would have been easily detected. We need to remember that the EEG remained totally flat for an hour and, specifically, during the time when the surgical instruments were taken out of their container.

The contents of the surgical toolbox could have been seen by Pam when the operating table was tilted up at a steep angle to reduce cerebral perfusion.

False, because at the time the table was being tilted, Pam was already deeply asleep from the barbiturates and had her eyes closed with adhesive bandages on her eyelids.

Pam could have heard the evocative sounds of the tools, which may have reminded her unconsciously of her father's toolbox and an electric toothbrush. Upon her awakening, her brain could have then put together these images buried in her memory. In the same way, she could have heard the conversation of the surgeon and the cardiologist.

False, because the pulseless electrical activity (PEA) measured during Pamela's operation was just as flat as her EEG. (The PEA indicates the electrical conductivity between the auditory nerve and the brain, which allows us to know if an auditory stimulation is correctly received by the brain.) This test is used to detect tumorous pathologies of the acoustic nerve and congenital deafness. In this case, the PEA allowed the doctors to follow Pam's cerebral activity, which was flat, as we say. Therefore, it was impossible for her to perceive even the slightest sound at a cerebral level. Moreover, there was no music, no birdsong, no noise of waterfalls in the operating room. All such visual and auditory perceptions originating in the brain would have appeared on the electric recording of the occipital lobe (visual area) or on the PEA.

As she was being operated on, Pam must have heard various sounds that she interpreted as music. The electric lancet made sharp sounds that were similar to birdsongs, and the circulation of her blood in the tubing outside her body could have sounded like a waterfall.

False. None of these sounds could have been heard by Pam in these conditions of cardiac arrest given that her PEA remained perfectly flat during the operation. The continuous noise that was transmitted into her ears in order to measure her PEA would, in any case, have prevented her from hearing any sounds from her auditory environment.

Pam could have seen the surgical instruments before she went under or at the moment she woke up and then believed that the perception had happened during her operation.

False. At the time of her going under, the surgical instruments had not yet been laid out near the operating table. In order to reduce the risk of infection, surgical equipment is not exposed to the open air until the last possible moment. That's always how it's done. Moreover, when Pam entered the operating room, the anesthesia had already begun taking effect. She couldn't have seen anything at the end of the operation, either. This is because she was only awakened much later, in a room far from the operating room, after having undergone the procedure to return her body to a normal temperature.

This single case of a brain death that was induced, confirmed, and scientifically proven should have been enough to demonstrate that consciousness is possible after death. However, we will definitely need to wait many years still before we can break the *omertà* that forbids the circulation of information that is considered to be outrageous.

From a clinical situation that is as exceptional as it is unimaginable, Pamela Reynolds returned to recount her journey to the hereafter. This journey is often foreseen in the minutes or seconds that follow the great departure. In fact, the man or woman who is about to leave this world frequently experiences surprising things at death's threshold.

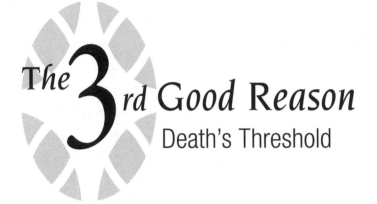

The 3rd Good Reason
Death's Threshold

*There is nothing more serious than to believe we know
what we don't know, and to defend as true what is false.*

APOCRYPHAL CHRISTIAN TEXT

THE BEHAVIOR OF
THOSE CLOSE TO DEATH

Resuscitation and intensive care services are the hospital departments
in which we observe the greatest number of deaths. The caregivers
who work in these units are witness to the specific behaviors of those
who are on the point of dying.

I have gathered here a certain number of common points from
most of my observations, arranged in decreasing order of frequency
of occurrence:

1. Calm resignation when faced with the imminence of death.
2. Feelings of serenity and inner peace.

3. Heightened spirituality; invocation of divinities; recital of prayers.
4. Euphoria and curiosity at the idea of discovering a hereafter.
5. Seeing magnificent landscapes.
6. Seeing deceased persons standing at the foot of one's bed.
7. Anguish and fear at the idea of dying.
8. Terror that is hard to control.

I am not in a position to quantify these eight characteristics with rigorous numbers or percentages because this list is based solely on twenty years of experience with ill and wounded patients hospitalized in intensive care. Although I have never kept statistics on these various reactions that people experience when faced with the imminence of death, just the same I can categorize them in approximate order of frequency. I have had this list read to the caregiver team in the resuscitation service where I work, as well as to colleagues who worked with resuscitation or in palliative care facilities. They were unanimous in their confirmation of how I had sequenced the phenomena I've witnessed. Most of them had already noticed, in individuals nearing death, the reactions I'd listed, but very few of them had ever spoken out about it. This subject, alas, is still very taboo in the medical environment.

To be clear, I should say that in the majority of end-of-life cases none of these characteristics are to be found. This is due to the fact that the individuals in question are apt to be in a very deep coma, which precludes them from being able to express anything at all. I would also like to make clear that the reactions mentioned in numbers 7 and 8 above—anguish and fear at the idea of dying and terror that is hard to control—are very exceptional. In the whole of my career, I have a memory of—at most—

ten patients who were in terror at the moment of death, no more than that. As it happens, I'm thinking now once again of a super wealthy businessman who, stretched out on his bed of pain, would lash out aggressively and nastily at both visitors and staff alike. However, a few seconds before uttering his last cry, his behavior changed utterly. He asked God's pardon as he wept the last of his body's tears. I can see once again his bulging eyes and his trembling lips mumbling this pitiable supplication. It was as if he had suddenly found himself in front of something huge and fearful to behold.

Below I have provided, from memory, a few reactions of dying persons that show a calm and phlegmatic acceptance as they face the imminence of the great departure. Fear, anger, and sadness are not present in the range of sentiments expressed.

I'm finally going to find out if God exists.

I'm going to be together once again with my parents, my husband, and all those whom I loved.

You know, Doctor, I'm just fine with this in any case. I've had my time here and deep down I'm not unhappy to leave.

Just a little while ago I saw my mother at the foot of my bed. I buried her more than ten years ago. She was in a halo of light. I really think she came looking for me. I'm anxious to see her—I'm longing to see her again.

For my whole life as far back as I can remember, I've always had a fear of death because I didn't believe in anything. Since my earliest childhood I've been scared stiff about the moment of my own death. I've always thought I would never be brave enough to face it. And now that I've come to this moment that I dreaded so much, I have no fear at all. I finally have faith. I am longing to be facing God.

The very *last* words uttered by those who are leaving are even more impressive.

I'm going. Oh! How beautiful it is! How magnificent!

This ocean of flowers that is moving toward us, do you see it too? You see it, don't you?

They're calling me. I have to leave.

My God, they're all there—all my ancestors are there. Thank you.

This white light—how beautiful it is! Never have I seen a light so beautiful and so white.

I have also received numerous e-mails from people who were at a dying person's side. Below are a few selected excerpts. The first story is from Françoise B.; the second is from Étienne H., a nurse in a palliative care unit; the third account is from Martine S.; and the last is from Pascal V.

When I went to see my friend in the hospital, a clear-thinking person who worked as a psychologist and for whom medicine could do nothing

more for, I saw her suddenly turn her head to the right to look at an invisible visitor beside the bed whom she called "Dad." Her father had died a few years before.

I noticed that quite often at the moment of death certain people say that they see, at the foot of their bed, relatives or friends who have passed. It happens quite often. I think that all those who work as I do in palliative care know about these things, but very few people talk about it.

When Mom died, at the exact instant when she took her last breath, she cried out, "André," while looking at the ceiling. My dad was called André. He died long before her. I know Mom well enough to be sure that the person she saw at that instant when she cried out really was Dad. She had a particular look when she would look at him.

Just before her death, my grandmother asked us to look at the "shining angel" who, apparently, was behind us. She was so insistent that, in order not to annoy her, we all agreed that we saw him just as she did—but in fact none of us saw anything at all!

HOW WE UNDERESTIMATE OUR CONVENTIONS

When we're alive it's very difficult for us to accept the existence of a life after death. In the West we grow up in a spiritually undeveloped, materialist society in which, by convention, from early childhood we are inculcated with the idea that death means nothingness. Or we could say that life, being closely dependent on matter, seems impossible when matter disappears. However, this is just a pure convention since there is no rational proof of this materialist belief. And I defy anyone to provide me with one! But there we are . . . our Western education, stripped of all spiritual values, has inundated us with this dominant, difficult-to-control concept.

We underestimate the impact of conventions on how we think, however, the impact is huge. Suppose, for example, that I tell you the color red is really yellow. That may seem to you to be false, ridiculous, and even absurd, but in truth, these selected words are purely conventional. Strongly anchored within our consciousness are ready-made truths acquired through a long and boring apprenticeship and transmitted through several successive generations. And if a piece of information, such as a scientific proof of the existence of life after this life, comes along to contradict what we've learned, it will be violently rejected by our unconscious. It's easier to reject the disturbing new piece of data than to try to integrate it into our body of knowledge.

This is why many Westerners can't accept the idea of a hereafter.

On the other hand, experience has shown me that at the moment when death seems imminent and unavoidable, we are entirely ready to accept another reality, totally different from the one we have always known and upheld—another truth that includes the notion of survival in another dimension. When there are only a few minutes left, the most assured non-believer becomes a believer, and the most convinced atheist calls upon God. This observation, made by numerous caregivers working in resuscitation or in palliative care, shows to what an extent our firmest beliefs can suddenly go up in smoke.

Leo and Gabriel

Our earthly life could be considered analogous to the life of a fetus in its mother's belly.

To illustrate this, let's speak about twins floating in amniotic fluid at the end of a pregnancy. Why don't we call them Leo and Gabriel? Leo is a materialist who believes only in what he perceives in his life in the womb. His brother Gabriel is spiritually more evolved and believes that a life different from the one he has undergone for almost nine months is entirely possible. They communicate telepathically.

Leo: Do you think there is life after birth?

Gabriel: Certainly. Everybody knows that there is a life after birth.

Leo: In that case, what are we doing here then? This life of the womb would then be stupid and completely useless!

Gabriel: We are in transit here so we can grow and be strong enough. We're getting ready for what comes afterward.

Leo: There you go—living on hope! All those ideas are just nonsense! There can't be a life after birth!

Gabriel: But why not?

Leo: Because nobody has come back to this womb after birth to tell us that a life exists on the other side. If nobody has come back, that means there is only one possible life and it's the one we're living here. That's it and that's all there is to it!

Gabriel: And yet there are many signs of a life after birth, things that prove that there are things happening outside of here.

Leo: Really? So, in that case, give me just one example of one of those signs you're talking about.

Gabriel: At some moments, I hear voices, noises, and melodious sounds. If you pay attention, if you really listen, if you concentrate and you think that it's possible, I'm sure that you too will be able to hear them. Since there's just the two of us here, these sounds can only come from a world beyond our own.

Leo: You poor fellow, I really feel sorry for you—your imagination is working overtime! In fact, you're so afraid that you're going to disappear at the moment of your birth that you make up stories to reassure yourself, so much so that you're hallucinating! As for me, I've never heard anything except the sounds of us moving around in this liquid!

Gabriel: It seems that when we pass over to the other side, we see a great light at the end of a dark tunnel.

Leo: Oh yes, you're talking about those NBEs—near-birth experiences, experiences at the borders of birth, which happen in cases of miscarriage. All that is complete bullshit!

Gabriel: And after going through the tunnel and coming into the light we will see our mother.

Leo: You don't say? So, on top of it all, you're one who believes in a mother too?

Gabriel: Yes, a mother who will take care of us and who will protect us because she loves us more than anything else in the world.

Leo: Come on now, think about it a bit, what you're saying is nutty! If this mother overflowing with love really existed, we would know about it! She would come to see us in this womb! She would show up! She wouldn't leave us to suffer like this in such a cramped, dark corner!

Gabriel: You are mistaken. Our mother is all around us and we are in her. We live and we move thanks to her. We exist thanks to her and to the love she brings to us.

Leo: Hey man, you're losing it! You're not going to be like one of those nuts who believe in Mother!

Gabriel: When we pass over to the other side, she will be there and she will take us in her arms . . .

Leo: But you're not going to exist when you pass to the other side!

Gabriel: What makes you say that?

Leo: It's this cord attached to your abdomen that's keeping you alive. Without this cord, you are nothing and no life is possible. When you pass to the other side, this cord will be cut. You'll have no way of receiving oxygen and glucose. Deprived of these two vital elements, you'll be dead in less than three minutes. Just look—I'll show you. You'll see what happens to you if I put a kink in your cord with my feet. Like this!

Gabriel: AAArrrrrghghghgh! Gulp, gulp, gulp. AAArrrrrghghghgh! Sssssstooopp! I'm choking! AAAAAh!

Leo: Ah ha! Bad boy—you see what you turn into in a few seconds without this cord. You turn grey all over; you die and you no longer exist. Ha!

Gabriel: AAArrrrrghghghgh!

Leo: Okay, okay, don't get upset. I'm stopping. I don't want to have a dead baby beside me, I can assure you. I just wanted to give you a little lesson to keep you grounded in the placenta. I have just proven to you scientifically that without this cord, no form of life is possible.

Gabriel: Wow! Thank you.

Leo: You're welcome!

Gabriel: I really thought I was going to die!

Leo: So you're convinced now, I hope?

Gabriel: Er . . . convinced of what?

Leo: Well . . . that without this cord it's impossible to live—just that!

Gabriel: No, not at all!

Leo: What?

Gabriel: I think that we only absolutely need this cord *here;* we won't need it at all once we're on the other side.

Leo: Whew, I give up! You really are a lost cause!

Gabriel: After our birth, we'll be able to move around in spaces that are infinitely larger than here. And we're also going to get bigger. It will only be at that moment that our life—our true life—will begin.

Leo: You're completely off your rocker! In the meantime, move over a bit—you take up too much room when you stick your arms out like that.

Suddenly a violent pressure is felt throughout the womb and Leo and Gabriel are buffeted around in all directions. They clearly hear a loud voice shouting, "Push, push, yes, yes, there you go, that's right, keep going, I'm beginning to see a head!" The liquid in which they are suspended flows away in powerful streams.

Gabriel is happy. He guesses that these upsets are the signs of a departure toward a new life that he thinks will be marvelous. At first, Leo is terrified, then little by little his tense face relaxes and lights up with a tender smile. He passes through the darkness of the uterine tunnel and sees a dazzling light.

Leo: Gabriel, Gabriel, can you still hear me?

Gabriel: Yes, Leo, only I'm hearing you very faintly. Soon we won't be able to communicate this way anymore and we will have forgotten everything that happened in the womb.

Leo: I think you're right Gabriel. We're going to meet our mother.

It's most likely that on the threshold of death, those Leos among us will also come to believe in God.

More Details about the Archangel Gabriel

Gabriel is an angel referred to in the Old Testament, the New Testament, and the Koran, in which he is the messenger of God. In the monotheistic religions of Abraham, God communicates with his prophets either through angels or by visions and apparitions. In Hebrew, *gabar* means strength and *El* means God.

He is considered to be the left hand of God.

In the New Testament, he announced the birth of Jesus to the Virgin Mary (Gospel of Luke 1: 26–38).

In Islam, he is known by the Arabic name of Jibril and it is he who revealed the verses of the Koran to Muhammad.

In an apostolic brief of January 12, 1951, Pope Pius XII proclaimed Gabriel to be "the angel who brings to human kind, plunged in darkness and despairing of their salvation, the longtime wished-for redemption of man."

Divine protector of all activity connected to telecommunications and of all its technicians and workers, he has become, quite logically, the patron saint of communication. (No doubt he must be watching out for all ITC researchers. . . .)

Gabriel's feast day is September 29.

An old saying announces: "Gabriel is the bringer of good news."

Prayer to Saint Gabriel

Saint Gabriel, angel of the annunciation, open our ears to the sweet cautions and urgent appeals from the Lord. Stay always close to us, we beseech you, so that we might really understand God's word and so that we might follow Him, obey Him, and so that we might accomplish what He wishes for us. Help us to stay watchful so that when He comes, the Lord will not find us asleep. Amen.

More Details on Saint Leo the Repentant

In the book *Miracles of the Blessed Virgin,* we read that Pope Leo, celebrating mass on Easter Day in the Basilica of Saint Mary Major (*Basilica di Santa Maria Maggiore*) and offering communion to the faithful, was taken by a violent temptation of the flesh when a woman kissed his hand. As the man of God that he was, he couldn't bear the violent and scandalous temptation that had overwhelmed him. In secret, and to avenge the distressing kiss, he cut off his hand and threw it away.

After that, people complained that the sovereign pontiff, now an amputee undergoing atrocious suffering, was no longer celebrating the holy mysteries with as much passion. Struck down by the disappointment he was subjected to by his faithful, Pope Leo called out to the Holy Virgin and asked for her mercy. She appeared to him, gave him back his hand, strengthened it, and asked him to appear in public. Saint Leo obeyed, and he showed everyone the hand that had been returned to him and told all the people what had happened.

Just like the archangel Gabriel, he became a saint who was the bearer of good news.

The 4th Good Reason
A Mind Outside the Body

As soon as I hear someone talking about those stupid stories of being outside the body, I'm totally beside myself!

ONE PARTICULAR "LEO" AMONG
A GREAT MANY OTHERS

OTHER OUT-OF-BODY EXPERIENCES

Based on the numerous accounts that come to me by e-mail, many of which I receive following one of my talks, out-of-body experiences (OBEs) do not happen only during near-death experiences. Contrary to what one might think, out-of-body experiences are far from being rare. According to the most recent study done in a general cross-section of the population, 10 percent of those interviewed stated that at least once in their lives they had experienced the sensation of spontaneously and involuntarily finding themselves outside of their physical bodies.

I generally refer people with out-of-body experiences to the good care of Sylvie Déthiollaz of the Noesis Center in Geneva, Switzerland. To the best of my knowledge, she is the only person who, with seriousness and rigor, scientifically studies every case referred to her. Subsequent to her studies at the University of California at Berkeley, this young woman—who holds a doctorate in molecular biology—created "Noesis" in Geneva in 1999 as a research center designed to study altered states of consciousness. With the help of psychotherapist Claude Charles Fournier, she has devoted a great deal of time and energy to listening to and bringing structure to people who have undergone this kind of experience. The work being done in this one-of-a-kind care and research facility deserves to be encouraged. In the recent period of worldwide economic crisis, Noesis, a victim of blind budgetary cutbacks, almost disappeared forever. This would have really been catastrophic for all those seeking wisdom and insights into the meaning of their paranormal experiences. Where do you turn and whom do you ask when the unimaginable happens to you?

THREE ACCOUNTS

For my own part, I have collected 124 accounts of OBEs that happened without any connection to NDE situations. Of course, to include them all here would make for a 600-page book that would very quickly bore the reader to tears, given how strikingly similar the accounts all are to each other. For now, I'll simply provide three very different examples of *leaving the body* that illustrate the phenomenon fairly well. After that, I'll provide the results of my research by discussing what the 124 accounts have in common.

---◆---

Case number 1, by Jacques D.

I am an osteopath by training. One night, I was lying in bed beside my second wife. Neither she nor I were asleep. I felt that she was worried and that her concerns were preventing her from falling asleep. It was past 3 a.m. and her sixteen-year-old son from her first marriage had not yet come home.

Feeling that she was very anxious, I said to her, "Don't worry about it, I'll leave my body and go looking for him!" In less than one second, I was in front of him. He was in a bistro drinking beer. I looked him straight in the eye and said to him in an authoritative tone, "Okay, you've had enough to drink, come back home right now! Right away, you hear?!" He was looking straight ahead as if he could see me, but of course he couldn't. I was totally invisible to him and to the others there and yet I knew that he was going to obey me. I returned to my body and said to my wife, "Don't worry, I saw him. He's okay. He's in a bistro but he'll be back soon." And indeed, after half an hour we heard him opening the door of his room.

Later on, during the day, when I asked him why he had come home so late, he said to me, "You know, Daddy Jacques, I was with buddies and I wasn't keeping track of time until at one point I suddenly realized that it was very late so I came home." When I told him that I had left my body to find him and tell him to come home, he burst out laughing and said that was totally impossible. But when I gave him a precise description of the bistro he was in and said that at a table near him there was a young couple having a terrible argument, he changed his mind.

That evening he came to me and said, "Daddy Jacques, I want you to promise me one thing—don't ever come looking for me when I'm making love!"

Case number 2, by Pierre Marc A.

I had an experience in the 1970s that really affected me. I was completely in the dark about the phenomenon that was about to happen to me. I was lying on a bed, stretched out on my back, when a shape that looked like my body separated from me, rose up slowly, and came to rest near the ceiling. My consciousness, my thoughts, were located in the head of this second form. I noticed that, without moving my head, I was able to look in all directions—a kind of spherical seeing . . . no colors, no sounds . . . but the feeling of experiencing boundless happiness.

I have no idea how long this lasted. Then this secondary form of myself came back down slowly and settled into my body, slipping into place perfectly. Once I recovered from my surprise, I wanted only one thing: to go back to the experience and to feel that infinite happiness once again. In spite of all my reading and my attempts to reproduce the conditions of this doubling—I learned that it is called "out-of-body experience" or OBE—I got nowhere. Nevertheless, I remain completely convinced that on this occasion I was not one, but two.

Case number 3, by Georges F.

Dear Doctor, after much hesitation, I have finally decided to pick up my pen to tell you what happened to me when I was under anesthetic. Please excuse my writing and my spelling mistakes. I paint buildings and I don't have writing training like you. I know that you're open and that what I'm going to write might be useful for your research. [. . .]

As soon as the anesthetic was injected into my blood, I heard a rumbling followed by a whistling like a rocket taking off. Then I found myself at the ceiling and I saw the surgeons operating on me. One of the two surgeons was a red-headed woman and the other was a man with small rectangular glasses. After having cut open my stomach down to the navel, the man with the glasses said to the woman beside him that she had not properly covered her hair and that a lock of hair was showing through on her forehead. She turned to a third person who tucked in the lock that stuck out from under her headpiece.

The anesthetist was calm. He didn't seem worried about anything at all. He was sitting still on his stool reading a newspaper. When I woke up, I asked him if he'd had any difficulty with me and he said no. I asked him that because I'd heard stories of what happens during NDEs. I've realized now that you can have an NDE without being just about dead—and even when you're in perfect health. What do you think of this? Please write me back.

These three examples show that OBEs can be produced intentionally and in a controlled way (case number 1) as well as spontaneously and by chance (case number 2), or they can be provoked by the administration of chemical substances (case number 3).

In all of the experiences I've described, the individuals were in no danger of dying and they were aware that they'd left their bodies. They were convinced that they were not dreaming or suffering from a hallucination. Case number 1 is remarkable because Jacques D. was able to describe the argument of a couple in a bistro located several miles from his physical body. The description of this original and unexpected scene demolished the adolescent's skepticism and, convinced of the reality of the phenomenon, he asked his "daddy" not to look in on him at an inappropriate moment.

Case number 2 is accompanied by a feeling of "infinite happiness" and includes the ability to see in all directions, as well as the sensation of "being two"—a mind dissociated from the physical body. This experience is very similar to the transcendental experiences found in NDE accounts.

Case number 3 is also very revealing. It's hard to imagine how a patient being operated on would be able to describe what was happening beyond the area where the operation was taking place without his being able to move around—in this case, above his own body stretched out on the operating table. The operating assistant, identified as a second surgeon, had her hair tucked in under her cap by a third person so as not to risk bacterial contamination. Not being well informed about standard operating room practices, such a situation would no doubt not have occurred to the uninitiated person (a painter of buildings).

WHAT THE DETRACTORS SAY

As you might imagine, I had no trouble finding colleagues skeptical about the reality of NDEs. I had them read these three accounts so I could observe their reactions and take note of their resulting remarks or arguments. Most of these colleagues wrote me back in an amiable fashion saying that they didn't want to even examine these situations because they seemed ridiculous or weird. Others said they were at a loss to offer any opinion at all. A minority provided the hypotheses and suggestions that I am reporting here.

"Daddy Jacques" wanted to impress the doubting adolescent who was in a bistro that he was very familiar with. As for the argument, there's nothing unusual about overhearing an argument in a bistro. That doesn't constitute a proof.

I don't agree with this analysis. I frequent bistros quite often and I haven't once in my whole life heard a violent argument happening with a couple at a neighboring table.

Being convinced that you are two people at the same time, as in case number 2, is a well-known psychiatric illness that needs to be treated medically.

With this kind of reaction, it's not surprising that people who have an NDE prefer not to talk about it with those close to them, let alone confiding in their doctors. Someone who dares to come forward risks being locked up in a psychiatric hospital and treated for a dangerous schizophrenic delirium.

In case number 3, the person being operated on was able to see what was happening beyond where the operation was taking place, through the "scialytique," which is a centrally located light that is moveable and has little mirrors on the edges designed to focus the light on the operating area. The unfolding of the whole surgical procedure, as well as the story about the lock of hair put back under the cap by a third person, could have been seen in this way.

This is impossible, since in order to see this scene in the mirrors of the scialytique, Georges would have to have been awake. And he must have been asleep, given that what he reported "seeing" took place right after the incision was made in his abdomen.

Georges could have been paralyzed by the drugs but not completely asleep, which would explain how he could see his operation in the mirrors of the scialytique.

This is also impossible because during general anesthetic, we always close the patient's eyes with an adhesive bandage to prevent inflammation of the eyeballs. If this precaution is not carried out, conjunctivitis will result in less than ten minutes. The automatic reflex of blinking our eyelids that all of us have when awake is essential to keeping our eyes hydrated, but this reflex disappears when one is anesthetized.

Georges, not completely asleep, could have heard auditory information. The surgeon could have said out loud to his assistant that her hair was showing outside her cap, and later George could have unconsciously reconstructed the scene as if he had seen it.

With this hypothesis it would have been impossible for Georges to know that the assistant had red hair and to know that his abdominal incision went right "down to his navel." These facts can only be determined visually.

These discussions about the three cases show just how difficult it is to accept an inexplicable phenomenon. Although they are upsetting and make no sense given the current state of our understanding, OBE phenomena are nevertheless very real and it would be completely dishonest and illogical to choose to ignore them.

FACTORS INVOLVED
IN THE 124 OBES STUDIED

Circumstances of the OBE

+ In 84 percent of the cases, the OBE was involuntary and spontaneous. Most often it happened in association with a strong emotion such as a near-miss of a driving accident, receiving news of the death of a loved one, hearing examination results, or having an orgasm, for instance. OBEs have also been known to happen for no apparent reason, however.

+ In 8 percent of the cases, the OBE was induced by general anesthesia, making it therefore involuntary but produced by the injection of the anesthetic agent.

+ In 6 percent of the cases, the OBE was intentional and induced by techniques of meditation, holotropic breathwork or prayer or by the administration of psychotropic substances such as LSD, iboga, ketamine, or ayahuasca.

+ In 2 percent of the cases, the OBE was involuntary and induced by the administration of psychotropic substances such as alcohol, antipsychotics, or anxiolytics (anti-panic agents).

+ 92 percent of the OBEs took place when the individual was lying down on his or her back.

+ Only 8 percent of OBEs transpired when the individual was in some other position: seated, standing still, stretched out face-down, or sitting in a lotus position or during a walk, a race (in one case a marathon), or a swimming test, for instance.

+ 96 percent of OBEs took place when the individual was in a state of deep relaxation.

+ 4 percent of OBEs took place when the individual was undergoing intense physical activity: a sprint, a marathon, a sexual encounter, swimming, a car rally, or a soccer match, for instance.

The account of a soccer player is so striking that I'm including an extract from it here.

I had just gotten the ball and had to outrun five players to score. Right at that moment I left my body and was able to see perfectly how

all the players were moving, even those who were behind me. I also saw myself because I was above myself. I was able to outrun the other five players with no difficulty since I knew the direction they intended to move because at the same time that I was moving forward I was reading their thoughts. I slipped through their defenses like greased lightning and shot and scored.

When I shot, I saw the trajectory of the ball in slow motion—it was fantastic and glorious. Based on this goal, my team made it into the next round. My sister, who is interested in your research, advised me to write to you. I did so because I adore my sister, but I ask that you not publish my name if you speak of my case because I don't want people to think I'm off my rocker . . .

Belief System
Following their OBE:

+ 65 percent said that they believed in the existence of a life after death and/or a hereafter.
+ 35 percent were not forthcoming with an opinion on this topic.
+ 0 percent said that they didn't believe in a life after death and/or a hereafter.

Quality of the OBE

+ 74 percent found the OBE pleasant and would like to repeat the experience.
+ 26 percent were not forthcoming with an opinion on this topic.
+ 6 percent found the experience rather unpleasant or even extremely unpleasant and wouldn't want it to happen again.

Average Age

The average age was thirty-eight for those individuals in the sample whose age was known (the age range was from thirteen to eighty-four). It would seem, then, that age is not a factor in the likelihood of occurrence.

Gender

Women comprised 78 percent of the study members and men 22 percent. But this weighting toward the women is not likely significant because, in general, I have found that more women than men are interested in this topic.

Socio-Cultural Milieu

The socio-cultural milieu doesn't seem to be a meaningful factor. A farmworker might be just as interested as a professional.

Religious Affiliation

Religion does not seem to play a significant role and, in fact, is rarely mentioned in the correspondence that I regularly receive.

Repetition

- ✦ 62 percent didn't specify if the OBE was able to be repeated.
- ✦ 25 percent have had many OBEs.
- ✦ 13 percent have had only one OBE in their entire life.

A Wish to Communicate One's Experience

One hundred percent of those who contacted me wanted to make their experience known, but a majority among them preferred to remain anonymous for fear of being considered mentally ill.

In summary, we can say that the experience of being out of the body, which took place other than in an NDE, is felt to be an authentic experience and not like a dream or hallucination. Those who experience an OBE are nearly always left with the certainty that they are a mind or a spirit incarnated in a body. I have yet to meet anyone who has experienced leaving their body who thought death was like absolute nothingness. On the contrary, most express clearly their belief in a life after this life.

As with NDEs, I have not been able to glean any predictive factor from my study.

HIDDEN-TARGET EXPERIMENTS

If OBEs are real phenomena and do not arise from hallucinations, a separated consciousness would be able to provide visual information about distant objects—precise details impossible to see otherwise. Some researchers have wanted to objectify the validity of movement out of the body in OBEs by placing hidden targets above hospitalized patients who are susceptible to having cardiac arrest.

On September 22, 2008, Dr. Sam Parnia, a resuscitation doctor at Southampton Hospital (in the U.K.) and the Canadian neuroscience researcher Mario Beauregard made a presentation to the UN in New York on their project called "Aware" (Awareness During Resuscitation). Their study plans to equip twenty-five hospitals around the world with hidden targets installed above patients before they undergo cardiac arrest as a result of very specific surgical procedures. The targets are plasma screens positioned horizontally on the tops of high vertical columns. Due to the fact that these wonderful screens are oriented toward the ceiling, it's completely impossible to be able to identify random images continuously displayed on them from the position of a patient lying on the operating table below. Completely impossible, that is, unless you leave the body and rise up in the air!

Currently, as far as I'm aware, only three hospitals are equipped in this way, including one in Montreal, and none have provided a result of any kind. My colleague in resuscitation, Jean Pierre Postel, clinic director at Sarlat Hospital in the Dordogne department in the southwest of France and director of medical research at CNERIC (*Centre national d'étude, de recherché et d'information sur la conscience*; National Center for Study, Research and Information on Consciousness), has also placed a hidden target in his resuscitation unit. This is a small screen situated in a box the size of a pack of cigarettes, which has been notarized as sealed and on which random images display continuously. To date he has not received any convincing result.

It's true that it's still too soon to be able to draw any conclusions given that these experiments have only been going on since 2009. It was roughly in the same time period that plasma television screens were installed in all cubicles of the resuscitation unit where I work. We got into the habit of keeping these TVs running all the time—just in case. Although in our location these screens are more numerous, larger, and more visible than at Sarlat, we have not obtained any particular account of a separated consciousness watching a TV program during a coma or subsequent to cardiac arrest.

From my point of view, it seems very unlikely that this experiment of using hidden targets will produce any result within the context of a classic resuscitation department. Let me explain why I believe this to be so.

Accounts Are Rare

To obtain the account of an OBE, the patients must undergo cardiac arrest (which, in spite of everything, fortunately doesn't happen all that often) and must be among the 18 percent who have an out-of-body experience and speak about it. We also know that only some of the people in this 18 percent are able to describe an OBE in an articulate way. This subset amounts to about 40 percent of the 18 percent in my study and between 30 percent and 70 percent (of the 18 percent) according to other authors.

Another essential factor must not be ignored: The person who undergoes an OBE rarely speaks about it in the days immediately following the event and will sometimes wait months or even years before coming to terms with the experience. And speaking about it to medical personnel is another step that is difficult for the individual who has undergone such an experience. It is certain that, in this context, the doctor is the last person they want to confide in because the fear of being given a psychiatric classification is still a huge disincentive that shouldn't be underestimated.

No Accounts of Seeing TV Images during an NDE

Among the hundreds of accounts of NDEs that I've collected over all these years, I have not obtained a single case of a departing or departed soul viewing televised or computer images in the course of the experience. This is despite the fact that some of these experiences take place in hospital rooms, in public places (cafés, malls), or at home—places where TVs are likely to be present and turned on. I have searched the literature and there too I have not found a single account that reported seeing images from film, video, or television during an NDE.

During one of my presentations, I spoke of my doubts about the efficacy of using hidden targets to show that OBEs during an NDE were not hallucinations. A young woman interrupted me to say that she had had an OBE in a movie theater when she suffered a cerebral aneurysm. She went on to share her experience with us. I am including here a written account that she kindly sent me a few days after my talk.

I remember very clearly the beginning of the film, The Big Blue, *but after that nothing at all. I had dozed off on my husband's shoulder. He wasn't upset because I often did that when we were watching TV together or when we were at the movies. I would lean on him in that way when I wasn't interested in the film or in what we were watching. I didn't do it to fall asleep, instead it was a gesture of affection when we shared a strong moment together.*

But that evening, it wasn't like that at all—I really did fall asleep leaning against him. I was very interested in the film but I had such a bad headache that relaxing helped. By falling asleep I had found a trick that stopped the pain that was crushing my head. I remember having said to myself, "This is great, you have found a trick to stop your headache—you just need to sleep for a bit."

I felt good—as if I had suddenly been plunged into a cool bath when it was really hot outside. After a moment, I wanted to open my eyes and wake up to see if I had succeeded in chasing my headache away completely (and also to keep watching the film). But when I opened my eyes, it was no longer the movie screen that was in front of me, it was just me. I was above my body and was looking at myself asleep on my husband's shoulder. I was up above the whole seating space of the theater. I wanted to let my husband know I was up there, and the other spectators too, but there was no way. Shouting and getting upset was useless—nobody heard me. I tried in vain to communicate with each person in the theater but everyone seemed hypnotized by the film.

I didn't give a darn about the film and I had no desire to watch the screen. I wanted people to know that I was up there and that I was able to see everything. The theater lights were not on but I saw everything as if it were broad daylight. I saw dust on the seats. I saw cigarette burns on the velvet upholstery. I saw the condition of the seats through the people sitting on them. I was able to do that. I only had to concentrate on something to be able to see it. I realized that the seat my sleeping body occupied was number 33 and I said to myself, "Twice my lucky number!" (3 is my lucky number).

My husband then noticed that I was breathing loudly, and he shook me to try and wake me up, but he couldn't. He panicked, stretched me out on the seats and shouted, "My wife is ill, my wife is ill!" People said, "Shh, shh," and others also grumbled about being disturbed. Then, after some time, they turned on the lights so that I could be helped.

This account shows that the comatose person had no desire at any time to look at the screen while she was outside her body—"I didn't give a darn about the film and I had no desire to watch the screen"—even though she had been really interested in the film beforehand. If, as she claims, during an OBE state the desire to watch a captivating film on a cinema screen disappears totally, we might well cast some doubt on watching random images on a surface one hundred times smaller and—on top of that—encased in a sealed box!

The "Visual" Perceptions of a Separated Consciousness Are Not Processed by the Brain or the Retina

When we watch a film at the movie theater or watch a television under ordinary circumstances, we have the capacity to perceive information coming from a film and projected on a screen or displayed electronically using a raster scan in a TV set. The information we're viewing turns into coherent images based on two physiological phenomena: the "phi phenomenon" and "retinal persistence" in vision.

The phi phenomenon is the visual sensation of movement created by the rapid viewing of a succession of images. The brain fills in the transitional gaps with the most appropriate image. Retinal persistence allows us to perceive stable images on a television, even though the images are displayed intermittently. The interruptions are multiple and repeated regularly at intervals of a few thousandths of a second. This retinal faculty allows us to perceive images without any flickering, presenting instead a crisp and precise image when we are watching a film at the cinema or on our TV set at home.

When someone is in a state of being out of the body and cut off from any cerebral or retinal function, it is therefore reasonable to question whether a separated consciousness would have the faculty of being able to perceive images on the screen of a cinema or a television. There is a significant likelihood that such a consciousness would be "blind," just as in the past photographic instruments were initially unable to capture televised images.

Absence of Proof is Not Proof of Absence

In our experiment with the hidden targets in hospitals, and given the negligible results to date, there is a danger that a lack of proof that continues over several years will discredit the accounts of persons who have experienced an OBE and, by extrapolation, an NDE. However, it must also be understood that, given the arguments I've just presented, it's entirely possible that we *will not* obtain any positive result. At the same time, it's important not to draw any hasty conclusions from that lack because that could be catastrophic for those who regularly have these kinds of adventures.

The experiment, however, is worth trying and, in spite of all this, I am continuing to leave TVs running at resuscitation stations.

You never know.

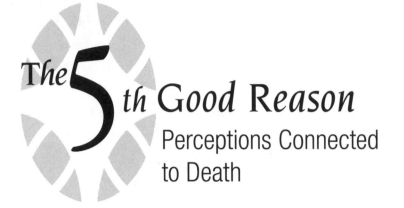

The 5th Good Reason
Perceptions Connected to Death

Those people who have seen deceased relatives appear at the foot of their beds were not yet in the hereafter and were not yet dead since they were able to talk about it!

ONE PARTICULAR "LEO" AMONG A
GREAT MANY OTHERS

A SHARED FELT SENSE

Perceptions connected to death (PD) constitute another major and relatively frequent phenomenon that strongly suggests life doesn't stop at the moment of death. Stories have come to us from individuals who were close by the person who was dying or who were at some distance away. These stories indicate that these other individuals experienced the felt sense of an energy shift—the departure of what we might call the "spirit" leaving the body. Accounts of this nature are not that uncommon; most of us have heard tell of such stories at least once.

It's very likely that if I myself hadn't physically experienced the "flight" at the moment of death of "something alive and full of joy" moving up from the skull of the accident victim that I was trying in vain to resuscitate when on duty at the Service d'Aide Médicale Urgente (SAMU/Urgent Medical Aid Service), some twenty-five years ago now, I would probably never have gotten interested in the hereafter and I would never have written anything on the subject.[1]

This very powerful sensation of the liberation of a spirit at the moment of death was necessary and sufficient for me to understand without any ambiguity whatsoever that life continues outside our bodily envelope long after our departure from earth. I often say in my lectures, "I don't think that the afterlife exists, I don't believe that the afterlife exists, I *know* it does!" And I know it does thanks first of all to this powerful, intense experience that turned my life upside down and inspired me to write nine books on the subject. It also prompted me to give innumerable lectures in France and abroad to defend the thesis of the survival of the spirit. This says something about the importance of perceptions connected to death! Regarding this connection between research and experience, Sylvie Déthiollaz writes very appropriately in her book about NDEs:

> I would like to stress by the way that many of those who theorize about these phenomena have not experienced them and therefore are looking at them from the outside. Just as a psychoanalyst must have undergone analysis, shouldn't those who study these subjects have had some actual contact with them in one way or another?[2]

The beginning of my book *La médicine face à l'au-delà* (Medicine Confronts the Hereafter)[3] is devoted to perceptions connected to death. This book was published in October 2010, the same year Dr. Raymond Moody's book *Glimpses of Eternity* came out. Without having been in communication, he and I covered the same ground except for the fact that his terminology is different. He uses "shared death experiences" whereas I use "perceptions connected to death (PD)." What *is* clear is that he and I are both speaking of the same phenomenon.

In my book, I tell the story of Dr. Jean Pierre Postel (the anesthetist participating in the project involving hidden targets at Sarlat) who, when he was present at his father's final moments in a resuscitation cubicle, found himself in the NDE tunnel along with his wife—who is also a doctor—and his son, who is a nurse. During the time that the three of them were at the dying man's side, they all saw the same scene: a mist separating out from the dying man's thorax. They also had the privilege of being present at the touching departure of his entity through the tunnel of light.

PD CONFRONTS ITS DETRACTORS

It's important to stress that these experiences of perceptions connected to death (PD) cannot have arisen from hallucinatory phenomena ascribed to hypoxia or various metabolic cerebral disturbances as the detractors might claim. The people who have these kinds of experiences are healthy in both body and mind and have not been subjected to any particular illness or cranial trauma (which is certainly not the case with NDEs!). It's remarkable to realize that the experiences of those accompanying a dying person may be similar in some respects to those who have come back from death. This is further rationale for discrediting the idea that the image of a tunnel (recounted by many who have returned from death) arises from a hallucination induced by hypoxia transpiring in the occipital lobe.

A Study of Sixty-four Cases of PD

In conducting a study on perceptions connected to death, I assembled all the e-mails sent to me pertaining to this particular experience. I ended up with sixty-four significant cases, many of which contain similar observations. It would, however, be tiring to read accounts that often cover the same material—the only differences arising from the different forms of expression and different personalities of their authors. Thus, rather than presenting extracts or chosen passages from *all* of the accounts, I have arranged them by their differences, thus underscoring what is unique to each one.

In reading these stories, we see that they can be divided into two groups: certain experiences that take place *near the deceased* and others *at a distance*. I have provided an example of each, beginning with a perception experienced by Marie Laure V., who was present as her mother was dying. This account is followed by the perception experienced by Raymond L., who was quite far away from his beloved brother when his brother passed away.

When Mom left for the other side, I was with her. That was my good fortune. I will tell you how that took place. As soon as I go back to that moment, I see it all once again as if I was there. Mom was in her bed. I knew she didn't have much time left. Her breathing was slower and slower, and little by little she was getting colder. It was early morning and I had spent the whole night in the hospital room with her. She

had been unconscious for several days. The doctors had decided not to undertake any painful procedures because her cancer had finally gotten the upper hand. She was just on a drip of painkillers injected from a large syringe that automatically and continuously was releasing morphine.

The day before at 4 p.m. the nurse had come by and increased the morphine flow from 3 to 8. She warned me that it was likely that Mom would depart in a few hours. So I stayed on. I waited the whole afternoon. At 7 p.m. I called home to say that I wouldn't be back for dinner, and then again at 10 p.m. to say that I was going to stay longer. Around 11 p.m. my husband brought me something to eat, a thermos of coffee, and a blanket. I used only the blanket. I couldn't swallow anything; I had no appetite. He offered to stay with me but I refused. I preferred to be alone with Mom so I could speak to her, laugh about the good times we had spent together, and cry too—all in complete freedom.

Because I was speaking with her; I was speaking with her using telepathy. I remembered you, and I remembered your lecture when you told us how to be with people who were dying or who were in a coma. What you said that evening really served me well and I can never thank you enough for it.

At about 5 a.m. my breathing became synchronized with Mom's breathing and a mist came out of my mouth. The mist became thicker and thicker and grew in size until it filled the whole room. I then heard a very sharp whistling, then a very deep buzzing, followed by magnificent music that was strange and impossible to describe. I thought I was sitting down but I found that I was floating horizontally in this thick fog. There was no way to see anything in the fog. I felt that I was moving very fast and that I was plunging into another universe that had nothing to do with the room we'd been in.

Suddenly, I saw a hand appear, held out toward me, and I took hold of it immediately without thinking. The man or woman who owned that hand was surely in the same situation as I because that person was travelling at the same speed that I was. Pulling on the hand, I saw an arm emerge from the fog, a shoulder, and then a feminine body with a veil, hair, and then a smiling face looking at me. It was Mom. It was her but much younger and in perfect health. As soon as I recognized her, she let go of my hand and completely disappeared. Then the fog in the room withdrew and I found myself once again, as before, next to Mom—who was no longer breathing.

I called the nurse. Mom had just died.

Perception connected with death *near the deceased* represents 66 percent of the cases in my study. Out of forty-two cases studied:

+ Thirty-one had visual perceptions in the form of smoke, fog, vaporous silhouettes moving out of the body, or luminous shapes more or less well-identified.
+ Eleven had physical perceptions felt as a breath (eight cases), a physical presence (two cases), or a tactile impression (one case).

The following is an account of a perception of death experienced *at a distance* from the person who was dying.

My brother was a pipe smoker. He always had a pipe with him. In all his photos he appears with a pipe. He had a whole collection of them—

straight ones, curved ones—all shapes and sizes. He travelled a lot and when he went somewhere he always had to bring back a new pipe as a souvenir of the country he had visited. Knowing how he liked pipes, people would give him one as a gift on the slightest pretext. He would always fill his pipe with the same tobacco, which had a very special scent that I loved.

My brother and I were very close. Never a week would go by without our calling each other at least once on the phone. Often at the moment I was dialing his number, he would be calling mine and vice-versa. One day, we arrived at the home of mutual friends with the same birthday gift that we each had thought was very original— a coat stand bought from the same store. In a discussion, it was not unusual for us to come out with the same words at the same moment. I have a multitude of examples like this, proving a telepathic connection between us.

On that day, I had been driving my car for more than two hours when, taken by a relentless desire to sleep, I decided to exit the expressway at a rest stop, breathe some fresh air, and stretch my legs before driving off again. Once I was out of my car, I felt as if someone had poked two fingers into my back as my brother would do when he came up behind me quietly to make me jump. I also smelled, at the same time, the scent of tobacco from his pipe and I had a very bad feeling of foreboding, with a sensation of my legs giving out beneath me. I looked at my watch; it was 3:20 p.m. Later my cell phone rang. It was not my brother—instead it was Dad calling to tell me that my brother had been killed in a car accident at the very moment when I had had that bad feeling of foreboding.

Perceptions connected to death *at a distance* from the deceased represent 34 percent of the cases in my study. Out of the twenty-two *at a distance* cases studied:

+ Seventeen people had an intuition, a feeling of discomfort, or a sensation of loss of energy.
+ Nine people had visions that were either particularly symbolic (in one case a crucifix, in one case a pen belonging to the deceased) or not symbolic at all (in one case an indefinable geometric shape) or simply an apparition of the deceased (in six cases).
+ Three had olfactory perceptions (in one case the perfume of the cologne used by the deceased, in one case the scent of the tobacco smoked by the deceased, and in one case the scent of roses).
+ Three had tactile perceptions.

The total of different cases of perception *at a distance* is higher than twenty-two because in some accounts several phenomena occurred simultaneously, as in the example given before where there was an intuition (which is typical), a sensation of loss of energy (fatigue while driving), an olfactory perception (the scent of the pipe tobacco of the deceased), and a tactile perception (of being poked in the back).

It should be noted that the sixty-four PD accounts are all from balanced, stable members of society with no history of psychiatric disturbance. In these cases as well, socio-cultural level, religion, age, and gender seem not to be factors.

Fifty-nine of these individuals said that their belief in the hereafter was reinforced following their experience and that they felt comforted in dealing with the pain of their loss. Five had nothing to say on this topic. None claimed that the hereafter did not exist. None thought they had experienced a dream or a hallucination.

The important points covered in this chapter are: The experience of a perception connected to death seems to occur more frequently when one is *near the deceased* rather than *at a distance;* when *at a distance* an intuition of the death is almost always present alongside other perceptions; apparitions occur but they are unusual. In the great majority of cases, this experience of a perception connected to death reinforces the belief in a life after death and lessens the pain of loss.

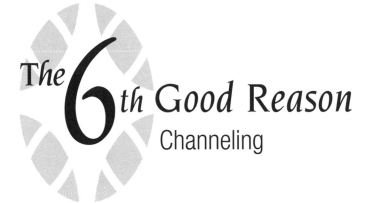

The 6th Good Reason
Channeling

When the day comes that a medium gives me the winning lottery numbers, then maybe I'll begin to believe in it just a little!

ONE PARTICULAR "LEO" AMONG A
GREAT MANY OTHERS

CHANNELING AND PERCEPTIONS
CONNECTED TO DEATH

The perceptions connected to death that we've just discussed in the previous chapter and the shared death experiences described by Raymond Moody can be considered channeled or mediumistic phenomena.

The term "medium" has been—and continues to be—so firmly bonded to fast-talkers and charlatans of all sorts that just using this word in a serious conversation right away relegates one to the category of crackpot or weirdo. Happily, things are beginning to change as mental attitudes evolve and the world of modern intellectuals opens more and more to the realm of spirituality. In fact, if we accept that a separated consciousness persists after death and that the brain is an emitter-receptor of consciousness, it's logical to think that the cerebral receptors of certain individuals work better than others to gather information.

We're not all the same in our talents, and channeling is no exception to the rule. In my talks I often use a metaphor that amuses my listeners: "We're all mediums—it's only that some of us are more gifted and more open to the spiritual world than others. Just as in capturing television transmissions, many of us have antennas— receptors designed to receive messages—and yet, alas, the great majority of us never connect them. A very few individuals are connected with enormous dish antennas towering over their heads—these are the privileged ones we call mediums."

THE CHANNELING PHENOMENON

In all time periods, human beings sought to obtain spiritual protection from relatives or friends who had passed on; some even spoke with them. This phenomenon is possible either directly or by using a medium as an intermediary.

Mediums are renowned for their gifts of being able to communicate with the dead in order to obtain information about the past, present, or future and also about conditions of life in the hereafter. Within the framework of a particular ritual, they enter into communication with the spirit of a deceased person and transmit to living individuals messages addressed to them. As in the case of perceptions connected to death, channeled information is received by clairvoyance (apparitions), clairaudience (voices heard), or clairsentience (physical sensations). These three types of receiving can be isolated, independent, or simultaneous.

We can say, for example, that the Koran, certain passages of the Bible, and the Vedas may have been received using clairaudience, by mediums who would have written down all these sacred texts as dictated by divine spirits.

Through a medium, a spirit may also manifest in physical phenomena—the most frequent being objects that move, such as the movement of a table, as well as the sound of knocks or materializations. Parapsychologists, whose thinking is based on spiritualistic work, classify the ensemble of these interactions of spirit on matter with such terms as "macrokinesis" or "telekinesis." Plenty of evidence exists to indicate that we can transmit an energy whose source is outside of our own bodies and that we can channel this energy to influence our environment.

Mediums play the role of intermediaries between the world of the living and the world of spirits because they have the ability to conduct energy, an ability that is highly developed. We also need to speak about "channeling through incorporation," which can be seen in certain spirit mediums. In this case, the subject is "inhabited" by the "visiting" spirit. Their physical appearance, the way they move, their voice, and even their facial features can portray to perfection the characteristics of the deceased. Most of the time this leaves no memory at all in the mind of the person who has taken on the incorporation.

We can also consider that "automatic writing" is a form of partial incorporation—the medium's hand is completely guided or inhabited so that messages can be written. This needs to be distinguished from "inspired writing" in which the medium transcribes information received in full awareness by the cerebral emitter-receiver.

CHANNELING ON STAGE

I have accepted numerous invitations to speak about NDEs for associations that are helping people who are mourning the loss of their loved ones. These occasions have given me the chance to be present at dozens of channeling sessions on stage. The medium who delivers messages to those present enters into contact with the hereafter by designating targeted individuals in the audience, either directly or through the use of photographs he has in front of him.

In spite of all these years of experience, I'm always flabbergasted by the precision of the signs of recognition, from the deceased person, provided by certain mediums. How could it be known, for example, that a mother tucked a blue teddy bear into the coffin of her child before his burial or that a deceased soldier is unhappy with the fact that his ashes are on display in the living room of his tearful widow? How could details as precise as these be known other than by contact with the entity who has departed?

I'll always remember the first time I was present at a channeling session onstage. The signs of recognition provided by the medium were so exact that I thought it must be a staged setup with numerous accomplices scattered through the audience. At that time, I too was a "Leo" (skeptic), as were the majority of my contemporaries. I was convinced that all mediums were crooks and charlatans—which in itself is absolutely stunning given that I had never in my life seen a single medium in action! This certainly shows the power of our prejudices and our preconceptions!

That was my state of mind when I listened to the performance of the medium who, in a flash, would crack open the edifice of my firmly held beliefs. The medium singled me out and said that my mother was tired and ill but that she would recover very soon.

That one's easy to unravel, I said to myself. Knowing that I was to lecture at this association, the predictor must have done a little research to find out that my mother had just undergone a gallbladder operation—a very routine surgical procedure that had been carried out perfectly. But I didn't count on what he went on to say: He gave me details of my earlier life that only I could have known—such as, for example, the first name of a woman I had helped when she was widowed.

Something in me was shaken. Could this be true? Could mediums have the ability to connect to some sort of database associated with the past? And could they really be in contact with the world of spirits, which is nothing more than a universe of information that's accessible at times? Could the hereafter really exist?

Today I no longer even ask these kinds of questions because I know that the best way of integrating all that I've experienced from being present at tens of hours of channeling experiences can only be explained by answering these questions in the affirmative.

WHAT THE DETRACTORS SAY

I know almost verbatim what people who denigrate channeling say. The arguments that they harp on about endlessly are always the same. They can be summarized as discrediting what the medium does and denouncing potential hoaxes that allow them to deliver their messages, while at the same time pointing out that they're making money at it. In general, these polemicists are people who know nothing at all about the phenomenon and who, for the most part, have never in their lives been present at a single channeling session—either public or private. It's therefore extremely easy to respond to them and point out the weaknesses of what they attempt to prove.

I need to make clear once again that many crooks and charlatans do exist, of course, within the vast brotherhood of mediums and that one obviously needs to be on one's guard against them. Nevertheless, one shouldn't jump to conclusions in mixing up the two; such evildoers exist in all walks of life, including the medical world.

Here are the principal complaints attributed to this fiendish work:

Mediums prevent those who have lost a loved one from engaging in their work of mourning.

False; completely the opposite is true. Carrying out one's mourning means to accept the departure of the loved one—it is certainly not to forget them. In any case, it's totally impossible to erase from one's memory past events that were full of love, affection, and friendship. I've seen parents, totally demolished by the loss of a child, regain their mental balance and give up suicidal plans after having received, thanks to a channeled contact, a sign of recognition from their cherished little one who has passed to the other side of the veil.

Mediums are all charlatans who exploit human suffering to make money. If they have really received a gift from God to help others, they shouldn't be paid for it.

I don't agree with this reasoning. Life is a gift from God. Our various and sundry abilities are gifts from God. For example, having the ability to undertake long and difficult studies to become a doctor is a gift from God. Should doctors then treat people for free? In order to communicate most effectively about the reality of the afterlife, one needs to devote oneself exclusively to this task when one has the opportunity of doing so. The best way to accomplish this is to do it full-time as a livelihood. People who claim that true mediums are those who don't get paid are people who rarely do volunteer work to help others!

Mediums are good psychologists who work the same way as mentalists. They shape their predictions and messages based on the reactions and attitudes of those who consult them.

False. You only need to attend channeling sessions to realize that certain precise information could not be obtained in this way. To illustrate this point, I use the aforementioned incident of the blue teddy bear that had been slipped into the child's coffin.

Mediums use telepathy to extract information from those who consult them.

False, because there can be information that is totally unknown to the consulting person at the moment of contact and is only revealed much later. The following account by Pierre Jouais is a case in point.

The medium insisted a second time, declaring, "The entity who is beside you is wearing a leather cap and aviator glasses and he is showing me a little painting of two big birds. Are you sure that means nothing to you? No? Well, it doesn't matter, keep looking and perhaps you will find something later."

And indeed, when I went home, my mother informed me that the watercolor of a couple of pink flamingos on the shore of a lake that she had in her bedroom had been given to her by a great-uncle who had been a pilot for Aéropostale and who was killed on a flying mission.

The information given by a medium comes exclusively from his or her own unconscious mind.

False, because there are cases of messages spoken in a language the medium doesn't know. This phenomenon is called "xenoglossia." In such a case, the information clearly could not have come from the medium's unconscious mind.

Xavier Bartoroki shares his account of a channeling session onstage.

The medium addressed himself to me and spoke a series of incomprehensible sentences, which he wasn't able to understand either. My half-sister, who happened to be sitting beside me, understood the whole thing. It was our deceased father who was speaking to me in Polish and wishing me a happy birthday. And yes, that day really was my birthday. . . .

Mediums who give information about the future that later turns out to be false are bad mediums, of course.

False. If we accept that mediums have access to a database of potential futures, just the revelation of that information to the person concerned can change what the medium predicted.

In the following case, Charlotte Gondais remained skeptical about the channeled information that had been given to her because of a prediction that she thought was bad. Here is an extract from her correspondence to me.

I have a lot of doubt about the power of mediums. I consulted one who said that this summer I would have a minor car accident that was not going to be serious. So I limited my trips to a minimum; however, the summer passed and I didn't have any accident at all. Now I regret having believed in it because the worry over an accident spoiled my whole summer vacation.

Perhaps if Charlotte hadn't paid attention to the medium's warning, she would have been less careful in her decisions and actually would have had that accident. It is reasonable at least to posit that this could be true.

The 7th Good Reason
Signs from the Hereafter

Signs, signs, signs. . . . I for one have never had a single sign! I'm convinced that the whole thing is stuff and nonsense!

ONE PARTICULAR "LEO" AMONG A
GREAT MANY OTHERS

INDICATIONS OF A CONTINUUM OR A LACK THEREOF

Often people seek me out to say that they have lost a loved one and are disconsolate at not having received a single sign from the hereafter that would prove the loved one's survival. They ask me, "Why do other people have signs and I don't? How should I take that? What do I need to do to have a sign?" I don't have an exact answer to all these questions but what I do know and what I say to them is that signs from the hereafter are everywhere because God is everywhere—all that's needed is to open your heart to be able to find and accept them.

Let's look at what Jean Prieur wrote in his book *Les morts ont donné signe de vie* (The Dead Have Given Us Signs of Life) about this.

> The sign, a bursting forth from the invisible into the visible, is proof of a presence when you think that you've been banished and are all alone. It is a support when you find yourself in the heat of an ordeal. Freely given, in love, it comes to us in secret and in silence. [. . .] Like precious stones, it is rare; it has to be rare. Given that the sign is personal, someone else cannot understand. Another person could not understand the concern, or the questioning to which it is a response.
>
> The sign instructs, advises, heartens, encourages. Heaven sends signs but they are not often received as signs because many of us are solidly armored. Heaven makes it possible for our night to be not too deep, but it does not allow us to bring violence against heaven. It's not a question of sending ultimatums to heaven.[1]

Opening up to the spiritual realms is therefore a necessary shift that we must undergo to be able to perceive signs from the hereafter. However, it's not forbidden to take a more scientific approach in order to sort out signs from the flood of information that we're ceaselessly bombarded with. Science always progresses in the same way: It tries to integrate an observable phenomenology by proposing a model of coherent functioning until a new element comes along that contradicts it. It's obvious that if we accept the reality of NDEs, telepathy, premonition, intuition, artistic inspiration, and channeling, the model of the "emitter-receptor" brain allows us to accept all of these phenomena. This acceptance allows us to demolish the fundamental principles of materialist thought that advocates as an unquestionable axiom the idea that the brain is a "secretor of consciousness."

In the innovative emitter-receptor model, the aforementioned received "awareness" would be a flow of information coming from one of four sources: a separated consciousness in the case of NDEs; an emitting brain in the case of telepathy; a field of informational consciousness in the case of premonition, intuition, or artistic creation; or—and why not?—discarnate consciousnesses in the case of channeling.

The following is a case that illustrates the telepathic power of a separated, channeled consciousness.

A BAKER BECOMES A MEDIUM
IN SPITE OF HERSELF

Philippe Ragueneau, who works in the field of press and media, is the author of quite a number of books that have nothing to do with the paranormal. In spite of his fame as a writer, I must confess that I'd never heard of him until a friend recommended that I read his book *L'autre côté de la vie* (The Other Side of Life).[2] In it, the author tells us about an out-of-the-ordinary experience: From beyond death his beloved wife, Catherine, continues to communicate with him as she had said she would when she was alive.

In the book we learn of statements made to him by his late wife. Some of them are troubling and upsetting, particularly when she invites her husband to tell others what was happening, in order, as she said, "to give hope to those without hope." She concludes by saying, "We revolt against all those things we are unable to comprehend and which are imposed on us. We give thanks when we understand and when we accept."

After being faced with this incredible evidence of life continuing on after death, Philippe Ragueneau agonized for a long time. As a man of reason he had to be very hard on himself in order to accept this bursting forth of the invisible into his life. Through the revelations whispered to him by Catherine, however, and through the support that she brought him from the other side, his pain of bereavement gradually lessened, allowing the hope of an eternal love to take its place. It was then that he wrote about his experience.

I was right in the middle of reading his marvelous story when an obsessive thought interrupted my reading: I had to send one of my books to him! And I did that immediately, without thinking twice about it or understanding why I had to. I will pass over the details of how I found his address with a disconcerting ease—details that corresponded, in fact, to true "guidance." Sometime later, I received a note from him. He told me the story of how, having gone out to buy bread from a local baker, he realized he had misplaced his house keys. The baker, without being able to say how the information came to her, assured him that his keys had been placed in his mailbox. This turned out to be the case. And also in the mailbox was a parcel sticking out that contained . . . my book.

Without this little episode, Philippe Ragueneau would not have collected my book because at that particular moment he was leaving for his summer place on the Mediterranean coast. He pointed out in his letter that the baker was the first one to be surprised by the information she'd given him. "I don't know, it's crazy. . . . Suddenly I had this sentence in my head and it just came out . . . ," she said to him, surprised at her own words. That evening he had confirmation of the channeled nature of this information when he asked Catherine about it.

Her reply? "I made use of the baker to let you know."

SEEING AT A DISTANCE

Information arriving in the brain is not always well managed, however. The cerebral receptor can sometimes receive messages clairvoyantly that, at that given moment, may be completely incomprehensible. Françoise Fulin was kind enough to entrust me with her story, which illustrates this kind of reception perfectly.

My twenty-year-old daughter and her partner were living in Italy. One evening, when I was in bed but still awake, I suddenly saw her in her apartment in Italy. Her partner was stretched out on his back on a sofa. He was holding his head and crying. My daughter had hidden herself in a double curtain at the window and she looked frightened.

I didn't understand the meaning of this vision and the next day I phoned and asked her what had happened. "Has there been an accident? I 'saw' your partner crying," I said to her. She replied, "Stop it mom; you're scaring me!" She then told me how she had been about to break up with her partner. He had caught her behind a very heavy double curtain, where she had hidden herself in order to speak on the phone with a man she had fallen in love with, who was pressuring her to leave her boyfriend! She was lost, panicked, and didn't know what to do. I, hundreds of miles away, had witnessed the scene just as it had transpired but didn't understand the first thing about it.

I never again had this kind of vision and now fifteen years later I am still flabbergasted by it.

ARTISTIC INSPIRATION

Didier van Cauwelaert is a novelist known for taking a position that favors the possibility of communication with deceased persons and the existence of a life after death. He has written the preface of such books as *La vie de l'autre coté* (Life on the Other Side) by Michèle Decker and *Karine après la vie* (Karine after Her Life) by Maryvonne and Yvon Dray. He has also included this theme of immortality in some of his novels, which include *La vie interdite* (The Forbidden Life) and, more recently, in 2011, *La maison des lumières* (The House of Light). Didier van Cauwelaert has garnered numerous literary prizes, notably the Prix Goncourt in 1994 for *Un aller simple* (*One-Way*).

Being interested in my research on the afterlife, this famous man of letters invited me to dine with him, just the two of us, during my trip to Paris shortly after my appointment at RTL Studios (a French language radio station formerly known as Radio Luxembourg) where, for a second time, I had been the guest of honor on Philippe Bouvard's program *Les Grosses Têtes* (The Stuffed Shirts).

Didier van Cauwelaert is a refined and sensitive man of great humility, and our dinner together was a totally enjoyable occasion. When I asked him how he worked, he confided in me that when he set himself down to write, he would remain for more than ten consecutive hours at his workstation without eating or drinking. During this time he would allow himself to be guided by a story line that seemed to come forth from his brain without his being aware of the passage of time. He would later discover that he had received a text that had been produced in much the same way as that of a medium practicing automatic writing.

It seems likely to me that many talented artists find their

inspiration through channeling. In this hypothesis, the information is not encased in the brain of the inspired writer but instead is situated outside of it. This brain would enter into direct communication with a field of information, the source of which is located far beyond our poor little neurons.

ARTISTIC GIFTS AND POSSESSION

Bodies of information received by the brain could also proceed from various fields of consciousness belonging to deceased persons. This would explain not only intuition and premonitions "whispered" by departed souls but also certain artistic abilities in the fields of painting, literature, sculpture, and music. A child connected to higher consciousnesses would be able, for example, to play Mozart with disconcerting facility or to paint the canvases of the old masters long since passed away. A number of such cases have been described in the literature.

Given that the consciousnesses of deceased persons differ as much from one another as do the consciousnesses of the living, the "spiritual sources" emanating from the deceased may not necessarily be pleasant or exceptionally talented. This transmission could just as well be coming from a darker consciousness and might transform the person in a way that is both spectacular and unexpected— for example, turning a decent family man into a rapist or a killer. Newspaper headlines regularly dish up these kinds of stories. Given that invariably there isn't the slightest bit of rationale for behavior that suddenly turns rogue, society seems content to condemn the guilty to heavy prison sentences and is frequently at a complete loss to explain what may have caused the senseless act in the first place. The simple analysis of a past background that was exemplary and virtuous in the case of a pedophile, a murderer, or a serial killer should be enough to assign credibility to the phenomenon called "possession."

CRAZY HANDS

Now let's discuss another unusual phenomenon that may be interpreted to be a sign from departing souls. It's not unusual to notice that chronometers stop working at the moment of death. Watches, clocks, pendulum clocks, and alarm clocks have been observed to stop at the exact moment when their owner's heart stops beating. Most caregivers who work in a hospital environment have heard at least one story illustrating this recurrent phenomenon.

My father passed to the other side of the veil on July 4, 2006, while taking his nap. He just didn't wake up. He was very interested in my research on NDEs, but he was much more skeptical than I about the possible existence of a life after death. Prior to his passing, we had made an agreement. Knowing that his heart was in bad shape, he'd told me that if there is a life in the hereafter, he would let me know about it by making use of the grandfather clock that dominates a corner of the dining room. And on July 4, 2006, at the precise time of his death, the hands of this wonderful clock came to a definite stop. This could be just a simple coincidence, but we need to take into account that it's more than just a little bit unsettling because this clock had never stopped before.

In the accounts of individuals who have experienced an NDE, we find, among similar descriptions, various portrayals of objects symbolizing the flow of time: an abacus, an hourglass, a clock face, for instance. Marc, who was the victim of a thirty-minute cardiac arrest following a traffic accident, tells a story about this.

I was in a light of love and this light was alive. It was speaking to me. I was shown my whole life, everything good and bad that I had done. My life passed by at high speed before my eyes in great detail and I was shown as an overlay the hands of a clock moving backward at dizzying speed. No one was judging me. It was I myself who was judging all of my actions.

Dr. Jean Pierre Postel sent me an account of a strange experience he underwent in the resuscitation unit where his father was on the point of dying.

We were with my son at my father's bedside when the hands of the wall clock started turning really fast and then they came to rest all by themselves at the position that indicated the correct time. I have no idea how this phenomenon could happen or why it happened, but in any case we were not dreaming since we both saw it.

I experienced something surprising that also involved a wall clock whose hands moved in a crazy way. On that particular day, a team of journalists from the French TV channel TF1 had come to interview me in the Toulouse operating room in order to make a short three-minute special on NDEs. The report was broadcast on the eight o'clock news on August 25, 2010. A few days later, someone surfing the Internet pointed out to me that during my conversation the second hand of the wall clock behind me was turning backward. I checked this right away on the channel's website and verified that indeed the second hand of this amazing clock was moving "in the opposite direction from how a clock's hands are supposed to move." The reader can verify this unique anomaly on the Internet using the date I've provided.

I also alerted Dominique Lagrou-Sempère, the producer, in order to find out if this special effect had been done deliberately to reinforce the mysterious or marginal aspect of the topic. The journalist was stunned and maintained that no one would dare do that without her knowledge because she was responsible for the montage. That this might be accidental also seemed very unlikely to her, given that it would have had to coincide precisely with the very few moments that the clock was being filmed.

After consulting audiovisual experts, I learned that there are automatic procedures for reversing images to make trademark names unreadable and that, in such a case, a second hand could seem to turn counterclockwise. But this explanation is not very satisfactory because any mirror image would also make the numbers on the dial appear backward as well and that was not the case here. So, if this phenomenon wasn't due to a cinematographic alteration, we have to accept that the second hand of the wall clock in the operating room really did move backward during my interview on that day.

Why?

How?

It's not hard to agree that we are still very far from holding the keys and knowledge that would allow us to answer these questions with any degree of satisfaction. But perhaps one day. . . . Without falling into the trap of seeing signs of the hereafter everywhere, we need to accept them as acts of grace when they do happen, without necessarily understanding precisely how they occur.

CONSCIOUSNESS TRANSMITTED BY PHONE

Messages from those passed on sometimes arrive directly by phone. Marie Hélène is a schoolteacher in a little village in the south of France. She has her feet on the ground and what she has to say is sensible. Here is an extract from an e-mail she sent me.

Within six weeks, an extremely aggressive leukemia carried off my husband, Francis, at the age of thirty-eight. . . . We were madly in love. He left behind a widow of thirty-six and an eight-year-old daughter. While holding vigil for his death, we had gathered in the kitchen with Mother to make coffee. When I heard the telephone ring, I went to pick it up, wondering who on Earth could be calling in the middle of the night. I then came back to the kitchen totally floored by what I had just heard.

Mother noticed and asked me, "Who was it? What's wrong? You're completely white." I chose to say that it was a mistake and that I was a little tired but, in fact, it was Francis that I had just heard at the other end of the call—my husband, Francis, saying to me, "I've arrived, little puppy." I recognized him right away. It was him. He used that intimate name with me when he snuggled up against me so we could fall asleep curled up together. At these times he would say to me, "You're my little puppy." He often traveled for work and as soon as he would arrive at his destination, he would call me and say, "I've arrived, little puppy."

If someone had told me that one day I would write down this story—a story I didn't want to tell to my mother or to a doctor—I would never have believed them. But having read what you have written I begin to understand that the "soul" or "spirit" leaves the body at the moment of death and that Francis' lifeless body, which was lying on the bed in our bedroom that night, was nothing more than an empty envelope, as you have said so clearly in your books.

This stunning account that suggests that telephone communication is possible following a death would not shock my colleague Dr. John Lerma who worked for ten years in a palliative care unit at the Houston Medical Center. And he has good reason not to be shocked: He witnessed this strange phenomenon with one of his patients! The episode is related in his book *Into the Light*.[3]

Dr. Lerma had been aware for a few hours of the death of Mary Esther, who had been hospitalized in his facility in room 236. He was getting ready to tell Isaac, the old lady's son, that his mother had passed on, when a mysterious call came in to the nurses' station. As Dr. Lerma explains . . .

A few hours after her death, I was at the nursing station to see if they had managed to contact Mary Esther's son, when the phone began to ring. The call display indicated that the call was coming from room 236. The nurse picked up the phone, wondering who could be calling from that room. She said, "Can I help you?" She thought that perhaps Isaac had come into the room without her noticing. She listened for a

moment and at first seemed confused, then frightened. She handed me
the phone and gestured for me to listen. Putting the receiver to my ear,
I heard a distant, clear voice saying, "Tell my son that I'm okay. Tell my
son that I'm okay." The sentence was repeated several times and then
the line fell silent. The nurse said, "Did you hear that? Was that Mary
Esther? It certainly was Mary Esther's voice."

The nurse and Dr. Lerma rushed to room 236 and found that
Mary Esther was definitely there, in her bed, dead. Of course, the
old lady had not moved an inch and she was as cold and stiff as anyone who has been dead for a few hours. She certainly could not have
made that call and there was no one else in the room. The doctor
made clear that, "If someone had left room 236 after making this call
we would have seen them from the nursing station."

But the story doesn't end there! Another surprise was waiting
for Dr. Lerma. About a half hour after this call, finally told of his
mother's death, Isaac arrived in the facility and asked the doctor if
someone had helped his mother hold the phone receiver so she could
call him. Those looking after Mary Esther knew that she was much
too weak to make that kind of effort so the assumption her son
made seemed logical. When the doctor asked why he was asking the
question, Isaac replied, "Please don't think I'm crazy, but I received
a telephone call from my mother telling me she was okay. She didn't
answer when I spoke and then the line went dead. When I tried to
call the nursing station, no one answered." Dr. Lerma was stunned
because when Isaac had received this call, Mary Esther had been dead
for a long time!

Dr. Melvin Morse is a U.S. pediatrician well known for his

research on NDEs in children. I was pleased to meet this illustrious doctor in Belgium where we both had been invited to lecture at the convention center in Liège. I very soon realized that, like most great men, Dr. Morse is a very warm and humble person. We quickly fell into an exciting conversation on the topic of survival after death and on the status of our respective research in this area. Just as had happened to me while I was in emergency medicine, this NDE specialist had undergone a personal experience that turned his view of the "afterlife" upside down.

His father appeared to him in the middle of the night after he had disconnected his phone following a long and arduous day of work. Melvin's dad appeared to tell him to check his messages because there was something important he needed to hear. Without the slightest hesitation, or the slightest doubt about this mind-boggling apparition, Dr. Morse immediately complied and then . . . what a surprise! There was indeed a recorded message, most urgently asking Melvin to contact his mother.

The doctor's mother then immediately told him that his father had just died!

HELLO! FROM WHERE? AH! FROM OVER THERE!

Father François Brune is known worldwide for his research work on a really unique discipline by the name of Instrumental Trans-Communication (ITC). For most of our contemporaries, this science, which consists of trying to communicate with the deceased by recording their voice, is totally unknown. It is used, however, by thousands of individuals all over the world. According to Father Brune, this unique method of relating to the hereafter could be being studied in great secrecy by research teams at the Vatican in Rome.

When I learned about the existence of ITC, I initially thought, like any "Leo" worthy of the name, that it was an absolute farce restricted to a bunch of very naïve people or charlatans. Today I have radically changed my opinion because I've undergone a series of upsetting experiences that have led me to think that under very special conditions, the consciousness of the departed can indeed speak to us.

In fact, the results of my research on the afterlife, which presents consciousness as a separated body of information that leaves the body at the moment of death, is not at all in conflict with this possibility of communication. On the contrary, as we've seen before, once consciousness has separated from the organic part of the deceased, it can perfectly well express itself through the receptive brain of a medium. Therefore, there is nothing shocking about an energetic transmission essentially made up of vibratory waves being able to make use of either an acoustic medium for the production of voice or an electronic visual relay used to synthesize "ghost images."

In fact, to the great surprise of those to whom they are directed, very recognizable portraits of the deceased sometimes appear on TV screens. This was the case for Friedrich Jürgenson of Sweden, one of the main proponents of ITC, and also for the famous movie actress Romy Schneider, both of whom appeared very clearly in this way after their death. The images received are striking and unequivocal and can be seen on most of the Internet sites that deal with this topic. Utilizing ITC, the clairaudience or clairvoyance of channeled information can clearly be translated into recorded sounds or televised images. Could anything be more logical?

Before having my first experience with ITC, I had met people who regularly utilized this technology. These individuals belonged to various organizations devoted to helping those mourning the death of a loved one. I also had the privilege of running into Father Brune, with whom I immediately felt at ease. In fact, how could one not help feeling admiration and a deep respect for this polyglot nonagenarian who, in spite of his impressive scientific and theological training, has retained an exceptional humility when faced with the inexplicable? With extreme gentleness and kindness, and with a great deal of simplicity and enthusiasm, this man continues to share the results of his long years of research more or less everywhere on the planet.

According to him, there is no need to have any doubt: The voices recorded during ITC sessions are really those of our dear departed ones who are speaking to us from a hereafter that, in the end, is not all that inaccessible. Father Brune's book *Les morts nous parlent* (The Dead Speak to Us) has become a reference book on this subject and a bestselling success that has been translated into several languages.[4]

Other individuals in France—including Christophe Barbé, Yves Lines, Jacques and Monique Blanc-Garin, and Monique Simonet—are interested in this topic and also work for organizations[5] that aim to help those who are suffering and in mourning. Their work has, however, remained marginal—in contrast to researchers in other countries more advanced in this area, such as Germany and Italy, for example.

But let's return to my story. On the day in question, Father Brune phoned to ask me to attend an ITC session that he was organizing with his sister in Caen in order to make contact with their brother who had recently passed away. To my great regret, I had to decline his invitation because I had a non-refundable, non-exchangeable plane ticket to a different destination. But then something incredible happened in the middle of the third night after his call. My sleep was brutally interrupted by the bedside table lamp, which turned itself on and off three times in a row even though its switch was turned off! At the same time I felt a pressure on my feet as if "someone" was trying to wake me up, and I heard a voice whispering in my ear, saying, "Go to Caen!"

I think of myself as completely "healthy in mind and body," and in recounting all of this I risk passing for a real nutcase. My wife, who was asleep beside me, was woken up by the signaling light but didn't hear any voices. Thinking that I didn't really have any choice in such circumstances, I canceled my planned trip in order to go to this incredible meeting with Father Brune and his sister. Apparently, I had received an "amazingly good invitation from the hereafter" as Father Brune said to me when he heard my story. It was an invitation that I couldn't refuse.

I'm going to skip lightly over the exact unfolding of the experience itself, which took place on January 28, 2007, at Caen, because it has already been told point by point and in detail in my book *Les preuves scientifiques d'une Vie après la vie* (Scientific Proof of a Life After This Life).[6] What I want to report here is simply that on that day, with a few friends and associates of Father Brune, we were able to record on a little sound recorder via a radio station in the shortwave frequency range answers from a deceased person to the questions asked of him! It was mind-boggling, staggering, and disturbing. I'm short on adjectives to describe that moment; just mentioning it is enough to give me goose bumps. Yes, from the other side of death, Father François Brune's brother was able to answer all of our questions! His words were perfectly audible and the expressions he used were recognized by those close to him as really being his. Since then I have been present at numerous ITC sessions, some of which have allowed me to enter into contact with my father who died July 4, 2006.

WHAT THE DETRACTORS SAY

There is no choice but to accept that the most categorical and acerbic detractors of the ITC phenomena for the most part have never once in their lives been present at a single ITC session. They're so opposed to the idea of it that they won't even venture to experience it for themselves to ascertain if it may be valid or not. I was more or less of the same opinion as these fierce opponents before my first contacts with channeling and ITC. Even though I was totally ignorant and had no experience with these issues, I'd nevertheless developed a very negative feeling about them. I didn't believe for a second that any kind of dialogue with the hereafter would be possible for the good and simple reason that I thought such a thing could never happen. This is a pretty feeble argument, I grant you. This stupid belief haunts me today because it was based on no tangible proof and therefore on not one shred of common sense.

Nevertheless, certain detractors try to discredit ITC by attempting to show that the recorded voices have some source other than the hereafter. As we'll see, their arguments crumble in the face of logic. This is a logic that's supported by the results of various studies conducted in research centers—notably in the electroacoustic laboratory in Bologna, Italy. Here's what the detractors have to say.

The voices received are, in fact, made up of random noise that randomly suggests certain words. These words linked together randomly make up sentences and, finally, these sentences happen to relate to the questions asked.

Although I'm not a statistician, I imagine that the probability of adding together this much random information in a short space of time—the length of the recordings rarely being more than a few tens of minutes—must be about as unlikely as finding a spiritually awakened materialistic scientist.

The words received in ITC are, first of all, suggested by a listener and then validated by other participants through a "group effect." The listener who generated the information then claims that you need to have a trained ear to decipher the message that has become clear to everyone once spoken aloud.

This contention does not hold up because, most often, several participants simultaneously hear the same message without any prior consultation having been possible.

Our brain is in love with logic and when it finds a solution, the illusion is validated as being reality. So if a written message is suggested before someone listens to the sound recording in which this same message is reproduced, the person will immediately recognize it. Lacking visual information, the person will never hear the message.

It's true, of course, that for those whose views are quite circumscribed, the recognition of messages seems much clearer if the information is made available beforehand (either visually or audibly). Conversely, it can't be denied that having practice in listening to the recordings improves the ability to hear them clearly. I've seen that those who have been practicing ITC for several years simultaneously come up with one and the same message while listening to the same recording. In such a case, "suggestibility" does not come into play.

The recorded voices are human voices coming from radio transmissions picked up randomly.

Impossible. The human voice ranges from 80 hertz at the lowest to 400 hertz at the highest, whereas those received in ITC can go beyond 1400 hertz—that is, vibratory frequencies that human vocal cords could never have produced. In addition, radio transmissions picked up at random could never provide valid answers to the precise questions that are asked in an ITC session.

Because these voices have never been analyzed, it's impossible to know if they come from the deceased.

False. Some of the voices received by ITC have been analyzed. Their characteristics have been shown to be 90 percent the same as those recorded when the person was alive.

The ITC recorded voices are an obvious example of trickery. Using a computer anyone should easily be able to "manufacture" this kind of voice.

False. According to the most advanced computer specialists, a certain number of the "feats" of ITC are impossible to produce using the most advanced software in the world. Specifically:

+ The creation of "reversed voices," which are different messages that are clearly audible when the recording is played forward and then backward. We asked Dr. Augusto Beresawkas of São Paulo University how, technically speaking, a reverse voice could be created. He replied, "The principal explanation for the appearance of a reversed voice is to accept that there can be a temporal fluctuation between our reality and other realities."[7] Sonia Rinaldi, a Mexican specialist in listening to ITC recorded voices, is categorical: "At the present time, there is no mathematical procedure or software with which it is possible to generate, artificially from one voice, another voice on top of that voice, proceeding in the reverse direction, in such a way that both voices are completely intelligible."[8]

✦ Recordings received while the recorder was in play mode.

✦ Recordings moved around within the same recording medium—each sound recording with the same identical message.

✦ A recording being taped at a constant speed able to produce, in play mode, four different voices: an initial voice audible at the same speed as that of the recording, a second voice at double the speed, a third voice when the speed was cut in half, and finally a fourth voice when the recording was played backward![9]

✦ More surprising still, on December 5, 2004, at the Centro Psicofonia de Grosseto (Psycho-Phonological Center at Grosseto, Italy) under the direction of Marcello Bacci, voices speaking a foreign language delivered messages to a selected audience. These messages were heard on a radio that was turned off! During this session, the most extensive precautions possible were taken in order to avoid fraud of any kind.[10]

The voices that are received through ITC originate from "remanent radiation."

Improbable. Remanent radiation can be defined as information fields propagated from specific geographic locations.

Studies conducted by Sinesio Darnel help us understand this phenomenon. This researcher has shown that specific places have an actual memory that can be brought out through sound recordings. For example, in the ruins of a hermitage located in the principality of Andorra, we were able repeatedly to record recitations of the rosary at intervals some years apart. In another example, in the remains of an abandoned house in the Pyrenees, we captured the wailing of a woman asking for forgiveness. When we moved six hundred yards away from the place, the recording picked up nothing.

However, messages received through ITC are not restricted to information emanating at specific places since sessions are very often done at sites that have no connection with what the deceased has experienced. Moreover, the answers we receive refer to time periods that have nothing to do with the historical past of the recording location. Although we shouldn't abandon this line of pursuit, it seems too simplistic to be an adequate explanation of the results that have been obtained utilizing ITC.

The recorded words are influenced by the unconscious minds of those who conduct the ITC session. Electric signals from the brain are picked up by the magnetic tape of the recorder.

Since the information produced through ITC contains data that is totally unknown to those conducting the session, this is a very unlikely hypothesis. On the other hand, if it is true that the brain can transmit telepathic thoughts, it's hard to see how these thoughts could be initially decoded into words and spoken language before being recorded on tape.

AN INEXPLICABLE PHENOMENON

Dozens of researchers qualified in electroacoustics have minutely studied and "dissected" the recorded voices of ITC in a laboratory setting using the most modern means available. They also take into account the most current scientific data. The result? They are unanimous in recognizing that the phenomenon known as ITC is completely inexplicable. To my knowledge, none of them have been able to discredit ITC as a hoax. Indeed, what scientist would be able to resist the desire to announce a hoax if the slightest shred of evidence to that effect existed?

Along the same lines, deception by an outside party is excluded because the deceiving party would have to have known the precise wavelength used by the experimenter for listening. The deceiver would also have to have access to a powerful listening device and, finally and most importantly, would have to be able to provide precise information known only to the listener.[11]

Again, to my mind, the only rational explanation for ITC is an acceptance of the idea that our consciousness separates from the physical body at the moment of death and continues to live on in the hereafter. We will review this in the next chapter, which presents a conclusive summation of my findings.

Conclusion

A SEPARATED CONSCIOUSNESS

Based on what I've been able to learn by assembling the different accounts I've studied, I've concluded that things take place as if we have a consciousness that separates itself from the body at the moment of death. The consciousness leaves the body temporarily in the case of NDE or OBE and permanently in cases of actual death. From the other side of death, this consciousness is capable of providing information that may be picked up by a medium's brain receptors or collected through ITC by a variety of vibratory, electronic, or phonic media.

In this hypothesis, the medium's brain plays the role of a receptor of the consciousness of a deceased person by conveying sensory information that is olfactory, visual, auditory, or tactile. If we bring together telepathic phenomena with the phenomena of NDE and channeling, we realize that the brain is actually, as stated earlier, an emitter-receiver of consciousness.

A SOURCE CONSCIOUSNESS

In this hypothesis, our brain is continually approached by separated consciousnesses belonging to the deceased—consciousnesses that, as in our day-to-day earthly relationships, are more or less contactable. Indeed, how much better would it be to be connected to the consciousness of an ancestor who wishes happiness for us or to a literary genius instead of a killer?!

According to the same model, there should be one connection accorded preference—the connection that links us to a higher consciousness merged with the divine, which we might term "source consciousness." If our brains were all identical, in touch with universal and constant fields of consciousness, our behaviors would also be identical. But of course that is not the case at all. We are all different. This is made clear by the fact that the information provided by a separated consciousness (higher or not) reaches our brain receptors in a brief and sporadic way. Intuitive insights, premonitions, and channeled contacts are provided in the form of a "flash." Following that, the brain will process the message according to its training, its experience, its culture, its knowledge, and its spirituality. It may variously reject, deny, ignore, or forget the message, or it may accept, integrate, and analyze it so as to modify a behavioral pattern. A medium is able to prolong the contact in order to deliver messages from those who have passed on, and the same occurs for an artist who discovers within the message—usually without realizing it—a source of inspiration. A brain that has been possessed lets itself be invaded by a noxious consciousness.

Once we have accepted this model of how things work—the brain is an emitter-receptor of separated consciousnesses—the issue that remains is to determine whether or not our consciousness can be separated from the moment of our birth and during all of our earthly existence, blending at times with the same "source consciousness." Or is this separation only going to happen at the moment of our clinical death—in other words, at the precise moment when our brain stops working.

I would prefer to opt for the first hypothesis for the following reasons:

1. An OBE or a departure from the body doesn't happen only at the moment of clinical death, as we have seen in chapter 4.

2. Great discoveries on Earth take place almost simultaneously at different places in the world. This well-known, irrefutable phenomenon can be explained if we accept that several privileged brains may be targeted by information emanating from the same "source consciousness."

3. It happens that at the same given moment, a number of subjects can experience an intuition or an identical premonition or they may have the same idea or take the same initiative as if they had been directed by an identical inspiration. For example, two people might decide at the same second to do the same thing—buy something, take a trip, make a phone call—as if they had been influenced by the same source consciousness.

4. An overwhelming wish to make a certain thing happen can favorably affect several persons at the same time. Who hasn't heard this kind of thing referred to in the popular saying "Where there's a will, there's a way" or in the phrase "An iron will"? When we feel a strong desire to have something happen, people turn up to help us without even being asked. Can they have been touched by a source consciousness that

has been fed by the consciousness that felt this overwhelming desire? And besides, do we really know where the compelling desire came from?

On this topic, I have a personal tale to tell. In 1998 I was working in a small clinic in the south of France. I was full of the enthusiasm of youth and, like any professional at the beginning of his career, I wanted to change quite a few things in the running of that establishment. That year, the doctors in the clinic were preparing to elect one among them for the position of chairman of the governing body (*président de conférence d'établissement*), which had just become vacant. I secretly coveted the job, which would give the incumbent the power and the opportunity to update outmoded functions. However, I hadn't dared mention it to even one of my colleagues. Since I had been hired recently, I was the youngest medical specialist and therefore the least experienced. Besides, I knew that two surgeons were already candidates for the position. Even though I kept quiet about my wanting the job, that didn't stop me from thinking about it.

I didn't just think about it while I was shaving in the morning—I thought about it day and night.

Then one morning a colleague confided in me that if I were to apply for the position he would vote for me. The next morning three other doctors said the same thing, then four others in the afternoon. In less than five days, I exceeded an absolute majority—all without having formulated "orally" the least hint of my wish. The two other candidates got wind of my potential application and they were furious. I was elected with disconcerting ease and for thirteen years I held the position of chairman of the governing body of that clinic.

It would be reasonable to wonder who was steering my incredible desire that was picked up by the brain receptors of my colleagues. A separated consciousness? Maybe, but of what nature? A consciousness that is perhaps divine? Shall we dare use that word? Well, why not?

Marie D.'s account is a perfect example of this phenomenon.

When my mother-in-law died, I felt a certain serenity not only at the church but also during the following three or four days when I felt her presence near me, no doubt to console me. Then she was gone. I believe that we're all connected by a consciousness that is in us and around us. Otherwise how can you explain the fact that what I ask of the universe comes to pass and that I need only to think of someone for them to call me or encounter me in person?

I have a sense that there is a link to the center of my brain that, little by little, connects me to the hereafter, which I prefer to call the universe. I have read several books by foreign researchers to try and understand this, but I can't imagine telling my doctor about all that. What I feel is different from what those around me feel. I hope that modern medicine will evolve. Take good care.

There is one other strange personal story that might help support the theoretical existence of a separated source consciousness. I say "might" because it goes without saying that we cannot draw any hasty conclusions based on an isolated, anecdotal experience. However, this unique account is attractive because it could be explained using the hypothesis that we're proposing in this discussion.

On that particular day I had just conducted a book launch when a young woman came up to me to get her book signed. Below I have pieced together our improbable conversation from memory.

I don't regret having come to your lecture, Doctor—it was very interesting and I think it will really help me. As you know, I lost my husband just two months ago.

Really? But I don't know you . . . I didn't know that . . .

Yes you do. I sent you an e-mail through your website to tell you how much your book had helped me. It was an e-mail signed Fifou. Do you remember now?

Er . . . no, I don't think so. . . . You know, I receive a lot of e-mails and I can't reply to everyone. Did I send you a reply?

No. But you did much better than that!

. . . ?

Don't you remember your call last evening?

My call last evening?

Yes, last evening! You called me on my cell phone to tell me that you would be talking here today, barely thirty miles from where I live. Don't you remember?

No, I really don't remember that. . . . Besides, it's impossible for me to remember because I didn't call you!

But it was really you, Doctor. You really did call me to let me know. I recognized your voice immediately because I had heard you speak on radio and TV several times . . .

Really? And what did I say?

I was surprised about how brief you were, because without knowing who you had on the other end of the line, you said, "I'm giving a talk at Toulon tomorrow." Then you hung up right away. Luckily I recognized your voice and luckily it was I who answered the call and not my mother or my son. . . .

Later I did find Fifou's message in my inbox. She thanked me for my initiatives and encouraged me to continue my work. But she did not tell me her cell phone number. So it would have been completely impossible for me to have informed her about the talk that way.

Whew! At least I hadn't just suffered a transient global amnesia!

There are two ways of solving this mystery. Either Fifou is a hysterical confabulator—even though she seemed to me to be healthy in both mind and body (in my capacity as a doctor I can't rule out this possibility)—or her telephone line was connected to information coming from a source consciousness while connected to my own consciousness.

I don't have the answer.

But if there is something to the source consciousness idea, what if this source consciousness, fed by the aggregate of our consciousnesses, is capable of influencing people's behavior and acting on matter and events in one's life?

And what if this consciousness is capable of providing us with signs of survival beyond death?

And what if this source consciousness is what the inhabitants of this planet call God?

Accepting without understanding is the antithesis of scientific thought that, in fact, always tries to explain everything. This is the basis of the massive and persistent rejection of all that we conventionally call the "paranormal." However, we need to have enough humility to recognize that we are still very far from having the means of rationalizing everything with our tiny brains—so small and tiny that we don't even know how they work!

We really are something!

According to skeptics and detractors, the existence of a life after this life, and therefore of a hereafter, has not been scientifically proven because for them the experience of an NDE is a phenomenon that is observable only by those undergoing it. Coupled with this, what people who have undergone an NDE tell us about their experience is, of course, not reproducible in a laboratory or measurable by equipment designed for this purpose. It's hard to imagine a resuscitation anesthetist producing old-fashioned comas in a resuscitation facility just to "measure" the accounts of those who might be deliberately thrown into these pitiful states from an injection. Since these two conditions of being reproducible and measurable—which are deemed to be essential for a proof to be "scientific"—are missing, the hereafter therefore is not about to be recognized as a scientific reality.

Reasoning in this way, scientific thought becomes frighteningly reductionist in authenticating what belongs to the realm of the real.

For example, we know today that the birth of the universe arose from a colossal coincidence that is as fantastic as it is unlikely. In the beginning, the first elementary particles issuing from the big bang were subjected to two opposing forces: expansion from the original explosion, which separates them from each other, and gravity, which attracts them back to the initial situation of hyper-concentration of themselves. Had one of these two opposing forces varied by one billionth, balance would not have been accomplished and the universe would not exist. Given the probability of such a coincidence, the birth of the universe is therefore neither reproducible nor measurable. Because of that should we accept that the universe does not exist?

A public opinion poll conducted by the Association for Research on Value Systems (AVRAL; *Association pour la recherche sur les systems de valeurs*), published in April 2011, shows that 35 percent of those questioned in 1981 believed in a life after death. In 2008 this figure had only risen to 39 percent—a modest increase of 4 percent in twenty-seven years. Even though this is a slight change, it shows that advancement of our knowledge leads to an increase in this percentage. Believing in the survival of the spirit after physical death cannot then be attributed to simple naïveté based on a lack of cultural development as certain people still claim. In fact, quite the contrary!

Extrapolating from this curve, we could then expect that in 2089 the majority of people will accept that life continues after death. However, the progression seems, in fact, to be steeper than a simple linear function. If we accept the responses made by 521 subscribers to a popular science magazine[1] at the beginning of 2011, the curve could even be exponential. This is because in this new opinion poll, 64 percent of those surveyed, in answering the same questions posed in 1981 and 2008, assert that they think the spirit survives the death of the body. In this new opinion poll, 50 percent also state that they believe in reincarnation and 50 percent believe in communication with the dead. The progression of opinion favoring an afterlife in this survey was more than six times larger in just the three last years, from 2008 to 2011, than in the twenty-seven-year span in the sampling by AVRAL from 1981 to 2008!

Other indications are popping up that suggest a radical change of opinion about NDEs. Evidence of this can be seen in the release, in May 2011, of the first issue of a quarterly review entitled *NDE Magazine*, which is being sold in newsstands in France and in French-speaking countries. I made a commitment to publish an article in each one of its issues. The chief editor thinks, quite justifiably, that there is a sufficient quantity of news about NDEs to keep the magazine running. This indicates the enormous potential that people ascribe to this topic! (Who could have predicted even ten years ago that an investor would take such an editorial gamble?)

Eschatological thought is about to change its paradigm and we are at the turning point of this general awakening. Very soon our survival will depend on this reality being accepted by the majority of the inhabitants of this planet.

This is inevitable.

We have seen that there are currently good reasons to believe in the hereafter—seven good reasons to be exact. These reasons must gain broader exposure. Skeptics and detractors, generally through a lack of knowledge, often slow down the dissemination of valid information such as I have presented in the pages of this book. My wish is that my work will help those same skeptics and detractors make real progress on the path of knowledge—a path that is also, and above all, the path of tolerance and love.

Psychomatter—From Quanta to the Hereafter

Emmanuel Ransford

ESSENTIALLY, WHAT DO WE KNOW? . . .

I was delighted to read Jean Jacques Charbonier's manuscript. I found it lively, inspired, generous, and deeply human. It was heartwarming. Beginning with facts that invite us to rethink death, immortality, and the hereafter, this author sets forth a real message of hope.

This message will cause some people to ponder. Perhaps he will cast some doubt on their hasty certitudes. For others, who are in mourning or who are undergoing difficult times, he will bring comfort.

What of us remains after death? Many know that they don't know. They have no answers when faced with this important and oftentimes anguishing question. There are also many people who think they have the answer—the *real* answer, they mean.

The problem is that these answers differ and are often

incompatible. So, who to believe? What to believe? Where is the proof?

Today, the dominant materialism of our societies wants us to believe that reason "proves" that we are mortal and that nothing of who we are will survive our passing for any length of time. But let's be clear: this is nothing but a belief. Reason doesn't necessitate materialism, which is just one unproven hypothesis among so many others.

In principle, when it comes to the invisible and the unknowable, reason is devoid of resources and bereft of any way of knowing. It doesn't know if there is a soul that is stronger than death, or if, on the contrary, everything ends up disappearing—disappearing forever in an absurd drama of forgetting.

It is in this not very attractive context that, with talent and enthusiasm, Jean Jacques Charbonier offers us "7 good reasons to believe in the afterlife." Based on the strength of his twenty-five years of experience in intensive care medicine, which firmly establishes his credibility, he brings to light a host of disturbing facts that upset and throw into question our preconceived ideas. Certain of these facts seem to strongly suggest that death is a transition rather than an end in itself.

However, I will not be addressing here the question—so delicate and controversial—of the possible proofs of a survival after death. The reason for that is simple: unlike Jean Jacques I have no special competence in this topic. Just the same, I have been aware of several surprising phenomena around me. I'm thinking particularly of Magali, my friend whose eight-year-old son has already had two NDEs. This child regularly perceives things about people who have passed and speaks about them. For a long time, his mother put this down to illusory fantasies in a child with an overactive imagination.

One day, however, she came to realize the obvious—her son was not talking about just any old thing. He would mention exact facts that he had no objective way of knowing. From that day forward she understood that her son's statements were not mere confabulations on his part. Something else was active and continued to be active in this child: He is "plugged in" or "linked"—the exact words we use to describe this state don't matter. The important point is that he has access to information that he shouldn't logically know. He is accessing an invisible world where information is circulating and where it is archived.

Could this be the world of soothsayers, shamans, seers, and mediums—if and when they are not charlatans and other dissemblers?

Can we discover whether or not science can shed light on the question before us? More precisely, could it be that a certain reading of present-day science would help us understand death and the disturbing facts that surround it, such as those described by Jean Jacques Charbonier?

This is the question that I will be attempting to bring some elements of a response to.

First of all I want to emphasize that experimental science—unexpectedly—can come up with ways of testing the validity of certain accounts of people who have come close to death. I would like to take as a proof the project "Aware" that Jean Jacques has spoken about in chapter 4. Briefly, this project consists of hiding visual targets for patients who might leave their bodies (undergo an OBE) during a surgical operation.

If completely anesthetized patients really are seeing everything that's taking place from the ceiling of the operating room, then they should be able to see these targets. They should be able to speak about them and describe them afterward.

This experiment, underway since 2008, doesn't seem to have delivered any positive results, as Jean Jacques Charbonier has indicated. However, regardless of what the final result might be, what is important here is to stress that the project we have mentioned previously, Aware, by its very existence shows that certain accounts linked to death and to the hereafter are, in fact, testable. We just need to develop suitably crafted experiments that strive to exclude the possibility of alternative interpretations. I'm thinking of the frequent ambiguities with telepathy, which we know exists.[1]

Experimental science is not totally without means when it comes to "accounts of the hereafter." Science can invent means to verify crucial aspects. And this gives hope that one day, perhaps, it will have brought clarity to some part of the question of the hereafter! In the meantime, I believe that the afterlife is a topic that is too sensitive and emotionally charged for the debates that arise around it to be serene. So I don't want to engage in it. Moreover, we know and see all the time that "for a believer no proof is needed and for a skeptic no proof is adequate."

Exchanges between believers and skeptics are too often perfectly sterile dialogues. Neither one is listening. I would rather not engage than try to add to that. Given these conditions, what is the goal of this appendix? Its goal is to suggest, as a brief complement to Jean Jacques' text, how we might view the question of the hereafter from an unusual point of view. This point of view is a little theoretical or abstract and I hope the reader will not be too disappointed in it. It has to do with psychomatter, which itself has been directed and inspired by quanta, the energetic building blocks of matter, the small particles that make up the entire universe.

In the way that I have defined it, psychomatter is based on a fundamental reinterpretation of quanta. Quanta and psychomatter are presented in my books *La nouvelle physique de l'esprit* (The

New Physics of the Spirit-Mind) and *Les racines physiques de l'esprit* (The Physical Underpinnings of the Spirit-Mind).[2] What follows has been drawn from these two books and also from the following texts: "Au-delà et physique quantique (The Hereafter and Quantum Physics)" and "Qu'est-ce qui se trame dans l'invisible (What's Going on in the Invisible World)."[3]

The frankly bizarre behavior of quanta really makes you think. There are numerous popular books and articles available providing the reader with a bewildering selection!

FROM QUANTA
TO PSYCHOMATTER

Briefly, psychomatter is what you get by adding to ordinary matter a little something that is non-material—I call it "psi." Because it is very rarely activated, this "psi" is almost undetectable and is therefore invisible. Too elusive, it is mostly unknown.

Please take note of the risk of confusion between psi and "psi"! In quantum mechanics, it is actually conventional to call the packet of waves or the wave function—also called the "vector state"— associated with a particle psi (designated by the Greek letter ψ). The "psi" we are speaking about here is something completely different. It refers to a hidden, non-material content of the world, which, however, leaves traces in matter. (These traces are the indirect proof of its existence.) To learn more about it, please refer to what follows and to the list of books referenced.

I would like to make clear that the hypothesis of psychomatter is theoretically testable, notably in physics and in neuroscience. We should therefore be able to know, some day or another, whether it is valid or not. I can add that it leads to significant technological applications. These various points are broached in my two books mentioned above: *La nouvelle physique de l'esprit* (The New Physics of the Spirit-Mind) and *Les Rracines physiques de l'esprit* (The Physical Underpinnings of the Spirit-Mind).

Its non-material nature means that its attributes and properties are not those of ordinary matter. Indefinable and creative, it is not constrained by the space-time (relativism) of matter. Notably, it does not "see" physical distance, which means that space-time is meaningless for it and is transcended by it.

Starting from there, I adopt the hypothesis that matter is in fact psychomatter. So I propose that an electron is a little seed of psychomatter. The electron and, more generally, all quantum particles carry in themselves an invisible, immaterial, indefinable "psi." This "psi" gets added to its physical part whose characteristics we are familiar with.

Through this "psi," which is omnipresent in ordinary matter according to my hypothesis, the world of the invisible penetrates to the heart of small bits of matter. It takes its place in the repertoire of quanta. More important than that, it acts in the world through them. All this is rich in fruitful and potentially useful consequences—which conventional science can draw no advantage from today since it denies or is unaware of the existence of "psi."

I can prove that "psi" holds the key to the strange behavior of quanta seen in quantum mechanics. If we account for it as part of ordinary matter—which then becomes psychomatter—the "bizarre" behavior immediately has an explanation. Once within this larger framework, such behavior becomes normal and understandable quanta behavior, due to the action of "psi." It's as simple as that!

Could it also be that "psi," in part at least, holds the key to the mystery of the hereafter? I believe it does and it is this question that I'm considering at present.

"Psi" is indefinable because it is partially "endo-causal." This means that it's capable, on occasion, of making choices. These choices, "self-made" and therefore internal or endogenous by definition, make from endo-causality an endogenous form of causal law—hence its name.

"Psi" breaks the determinist shackles in which it was thought that matter could be locked away in solely concrete forms, lacking in abstract energetic abilities. "Psi" is creative and can take spontaneous initiative.

I would like to make clear that I am not unrestrainedly applying a naïve anthropomorphism to quanta! It's not a question of instilling psychology into quanta or their "psi." I hope this is perfectly clear for the reader.

I have simply chosen to use ordinary words ("choice," "decision," "initiative" . . .) for convenience and to avoid obscure neologisms, hoping this will not lead to confusion. The possible choices that get made by the "psi" of an electron have nothing to do with the decisions that we make throughout our lives. They are extremely rudimentary. The "choices" of the "psi" belonging to quantum particles (which, in certain cases, are called "measurement results") are very limited and strongly constrained. They come about or appear concretely based on evolutionary movements that are called "non-unitary," over the course of which quantum waves disappear. (These waves, in contrast, accompany any "unitary" evolution. They arise when quanta have choices, but their choices—such as which slit a light particle "chooses" to pass through—are unknown.) Non-unitary evolutions of atomic and subatomic matter include notably quantum leaps, wave-packet reduction, inelastic collisions, and tunnel effects. They have major importance: For psychomatter, they are at the heart of matter-spirit interactions that the dualists have always been looking for. (Two known representatives of dualism are René Descartes and, closer to us, John Eccles.)

As opposed to determinism, which is objective, endo-causality refers to eminently subjective content. The "psi" from which the endo-causality is emanating is of a subjective nature and relates it to the psyche. This is precisely why I called it "psi" ("psi" as in psyche).

For example, when an electron is confronted by necessary choices, its "psi" becomes active. It connects with a form of consciousness—tiny and totally negligible on this scale. The rest of the time the electron, strictly deterministic, oscillates. It is then a "wave packet." Its "psi," inactive and unconscious, is latent. That's exactly what makes it undetectable!

An elementary particle is confronted with necessary choices in the case of a strong "quantum threat." Quantum measurement is a case in point because the act of a scientist measuring the particle's actions determines that it must make a choice rather than staying in a state of all choices still as possibilities. (You will note that I am taking the example of the electron to craft the ideas, but everything that I'm saying about "psi" is general. This remains valid whichever quanta or elementary particles are being considered: electrons, photons, protons, etc.)

There is another very original property, burgeoning in consequences, that "psi" enjoys—that of being connected. The "psi" of an electron is connected in the sense that it can bond with or stick to the "psi" of other particles to form a shared "psi." Everything takes place as if each particle concerned loses its individual "psi," which merges into a collective "psi."

I call this strange property of connectedness, which resembles no other property, "suprality." It manifests through the presence of "supral connections," which bond together the "psi" of separate particles. This property, like that of the "psi" from which it's made, is unaffected by the distance between particles. Its existence today is firmly established and known as quantum entanglement.

A supral connection or a connection of suprality between two electrons, for example, is like an invisible wire running from one to the other connecting their "psi." This sharing implies that the decisions of the electrons are now unified and simultaneous, and they remain so as long as the supral connection persists.

This unification of two individual "psi" into a collective entity leads to a perfect correlation of their respective choices; these choices are no longer independent but, on the contrary, become harmonized. This correlation, combined with their non-relativistic nature (simultaneity, unaffected by distance), makes the existence of a supral connection identifiable and testable.

Suprality applies to any quantity and any type of quantum particles (electrons, muons, photons, neutrons, protons, etc.). It manifests physically through what is variously called "quantum non-locality," "non-separability," or "entanglement." This diversity of names no doubt reflects the great perplexity that surrounds it.

Up to this point we have seen just two essential traits of psychomatter: "psi" and suprality. Its other great originality is being a substance with two faces: it has two alternate states. It's like the substance with the chemical formula H_2O, which can be either water or ice. (One is fluid: warmer and dense; the other is solid: cold and less dense. This chemical substance exists also in the gaseous state, of course.)

In the case of psychomatter, we're not dealing with ice or water. It's either matter or "paral"—that's how I'm baptizing these two faces, or states. The first, matter, is present when the "psi" is latent and unconscious. In this state the particle has a perfectly deterministic behavior. It is oscillatory, continuous, and relativistic.

The second state, paral, is unique to psychomatter. It's present when the "psi" is active. For an isolated particle, the "psi" is "proto-conscious." It becomes more complex and endowed with changing scale, able to connect across distances due to suprality. I am using the qualifier "proto-conscious" to underscore that the tiny drop-let of "psi" or active psyche that arises in an isolated particle in the paral state corresponds to the momentary appearance of an extremely tenuous degree of consciousness—so tenuous that it almost doesn't exist. (Similarly, an isolated photon is not enough to make visible light. One needs to assemble an astronomical number of them for that.) In contrast, when a number of particles bonded together by suprality (they are then "supralated" or entangled) simultaneously move into the paral state, once a certain threshold is crossed, a real consciousness can emerge. I summarize this idea in the formulation: consciousness is supralated paral (entangled "psis" of many particles).

When a particle moves to the paral state, this event reflects the properties of "psi," which is then active. Consequently, it is inde-finable, discontinuous, and non-relativistic. The quantum relin-quishes its wave aspect to momentarily adopt a particle appearance. I will point out in passing that the famous wave-particle duality of quantum physics refers precisely to the matter-paral duality of psychomatter. (For additional explanations, I refer the reader to the referenced books.) I will add that the paral—or rather that any momentary transition to the paral state of a particle, which I call a "paral phase"—has an irreversible character. This arises from the endo-causal "choice" that every paral phase creates: It gets inserted between its "before" and its "after," rendering them non-equivalent. This irreversibility contrasts once again the state of paral with the state of matter, which is a state of totally reversible unitary evo-lution. We will see that any paral choice is, to adopt the famous expression in an article written by Einstein, Podolsky, and Rosen in 1935, an authentic "new element of reality."

After these unfortunately necessary preliminaries, I now come to the essential question: What connections does psychomatter have with the hereafter? We are going to see that psychomatter allows us to distinguish not one but two hereafters. There would then be two hereafters underlying quanta! That is, in any case, what we end up with in following the path delineated by psychomatter, which adds then two new reasons to the "seven good reasons" for believing in the hereafter provided by Jean Jacques.

The first hereafter is "near" or immanent. I call it meta-consciousness. The second is, in contrast, "distant" and transcendent. I baptize it the ur-after.

THE META-CONSCIOUSNESS, OUR NEAR HEREAFTER

According to the light that psychomatter sheds on the quantum world, the totality of all supral connections that surround every particle in the universe forms a gigantic network at every moment. I call this network "the great supral web." It is recognized by other scientific researchers as well. Ervin Laszlo refers to it as the "Akashic Field," and Rupert Sheldrake explains it through his theory of morphogenetic fields.

This web extends to the whole firmament. It is an immense web of interdependencies, of solidarities, of sharing, and of exchange—in which we all participate. We receive a great deal from this web and we give to it as well—generally unknowingly. Suprality confers to each one of us a dizzying reach into the invisible world. Because of suprality we become a supral "I," infinitely more vast than our ordinary little "I."

By definition, the supral "I" is what the ordinary "I" becomes when we add to it all the supral links that attach it to other people and, more widely, to the great supral web. Our links or our supral connections give us virtually unlimited psychic wings. With them, we are real giants of the invisible world!

The supral web, unobtrusive in the extreme because it is made of "psi," has significant practical consequences. It is a kind of telepathic web. For example, it is capable of making inexplicable healing possible, nearby or at a distance. When I say "inexplicable," I mean clearly in relation to the conventional hypothesis that matter is inert. In contrast, if we adopt the hypothesis of psychomatter, all these strange—or paranormal—phenomena become perfectly conceivable and explainable. In the present case (of a possible positive impact on a state of health), we could speak of "bio-psycho-kinesis." To know more about that, in addition to the books already referenced, I refer the reader to my text titled "Paranormal et microphysique: une approche par la psychomatière (Paranormal and Particle Physics: An Approach through Psychomatter)."[4] I will add that Dr. Larry Dossey merits special mention on this topic: He has extensively studied the influence, at a distance, of prayer on healing and well-being. Several of his books investigate this question.

The supral web contains, archives, and transmits information that is permanently deposited and added to it. This has been so since the dawn of time. Such information is called "supral information." Supral information results from motifs—of an infinite diversity—that are sketched or "knit" collectively by the supral connections that intersect each other as they follow their own paths from one particle to another. This information is generally unconscious and subliminal just like the "psi" that serves as its foundation. However, a state of great inner receptivity can help to hear it and perceive it. Meditation, which silences the sometimes-deafening noise of the thinking mind, fosters this state.

Supral information is an original and totally new form of information. It is this information that, in the framework of "psychomatter," holds the key to the qualia, the qualitative and subjective content of our experience. Supral information is encoded and stored—or remembered—in the "psi" field that suprality forms. Non-local and invisible, it generally remains unconscious following the example of "psi" itself. It becomes more or less conscious, in varying degrees, when the particles of psychomatter, which act as its medium, simultaneously move into the paral state.

A unit of supral information is the "suprel" (which is a "pixel of the spirit-mind"). This concept has numerous implications—enough I think to fill several books! For example, we might deduce the existence of various "spheres of unconsciousness," contained within each other like so many Russian dolls. One of these is the transgenerational unconscious of psycho-genealogy. Supral information provides, by the way, a plausible (and testable) solution to the enigma of qualia and declarative memory. (I am reminded that "qualia" are the perceptible contents of subjective experience. "Declarative memory" is the contents of our mental memory arising from our conscious experience.)

In the course of our lives we (our mind and our brain) generate a considerable mass of information. As imprints of our experience, most of this information then gets dispersed into the great supral web to which we are permanently connected. These traces of our experience endure there, perhaps forever, in that great invisible web and non-local archive.

Our meta-consciousness, the "first" hereafter, is then the totality of supral information deposited in the great web during the entire course of our time on Earth. This collection of invisible imprints is a kind of envelope of all that it has been our lot to experience—a lasting envelope, perhaps even quasi-immortal.

Our meta-consciousness is that part of us that will remain long after our physical death. It constitutes our "immanent soul"— immanent because it is very connected to psychomatter and its properties. It becomes inscribed in an immanent (or close) hereafter that is completely contained in the invisible dimension of our manifested universe.

Here is what I wrote about this in my brief contribution to Jean-Pierre Girard's book *La science et les phénomènes de l'au-delà* (Science and the Phenomena of the Hereafter): "Like a personalized 'immortal soul,' our meta-consciousness creates a form of survival of the psyche that each one of us has. It is this little piece of soul that belongs to us and that blends into the global soul of the world . . . for eternity, or almost."[5]

Incidentally, it can happen that we might sometimes contact the meta-consciousness of a deceased person. All meta-consciousnesses are, in fact, connected to each other within the great supral web. This means we can conceive of the possibility of a potential communication with "the energy of the dead" to use the expression of Arlette Triolaire.

Such a phenomenon, implausible within the confines of conventional physics, becomes conceivable with psychomatter. It provides a plausible explanation for the paranormal powers of Magali's son, which I referenced earlier.

My hypothesis is that this eight-year-old child receives and perceives information about the deceased through his exceptionally strong connection with the universal supral web that joins us together and connects us to our meta-consciousnesses. The fact that he experienced NDEs could only have reinforced and enriched this connection. (I will elaborate on this point later on.)

In concluding this section, we have just seen that quantum physics, interpreted in terms of psychomatter, allows us to conceive of an initial way of surviving physical death. This first level of the hereafter is that of the meta-consciousness. It is the eighth good reason for believing in the afterlife.

In pursuing this line of thought, we now come to a second level of the hereafter—a more "distant" level because it is beyond this world. I am now speaking of the "ur-after." It constitutes the ninth good reason. . . .

THE "UR-AFTER"—A DISTANT HEREAFTER

In order to discover and define the ur-after and grasp its relationship to psychomatter, let us return for a moment to what constitutes the fundamental and underlying originality of psychomatter: its endo-causality.

I would like to remind us that with psychomatter, every quantum particle through its "psi" carries one endo-causal instance. Saying, for example, that an electron has endo-causality amounts to saying that it has (thanks to its "psi") a capacity to choose or, in other words, the power to decide—clearly a rudimentary power. In short, endo-causality is a deliberate (or free) causality and is therefore endogenous. It manifests concretely by appearing random. More precisely, it manifests in a quantum indefinability.

In my view, quantum randomness is simply the visible mask of the partial endo-causality that is an integral part of and characterizes psychomatter. It turns out that this apparently innocent hypothesis has very far-reaching consequences. It can take us very far—far enough to touch transcendence!

This would be a good time to remind us of Albert Einstein's

magnificent sentence, "Coincidence is God's way of remaining anonymous." It is deep with truth.

In fact, transcendence should be sought in the direction of "ur-causality," which is an extension, a "natural" prolongation, of partial endo-causality that itself appears in the form of partial randomness or coincidence. Here's what I wrote on this topic in a text published in 2007:

> Ur-causality is pure or total endo-causality. It is not the endo-causality of psychomatter, which is only partial and limited by all the determining factors that control it. . . . Ur-causality abolishes the unbridgeable distance that separates being and non-being. . . . With ur-causality being and nothingness become . . . partners in an essential dance where everything is reversible—including the fact of existing and the fact of not existing. I convey that by saying that it is existable. [By its] "existability" . . . it is creator and self-creator. In short, the ur-causal is ontologically reversible. This crucial property means that it is able to turn itself into true nothingness (exempt from the laws of physics) and, equally well, to self-generate (starting from total nothingness).[6]

Ur-causality surprises us. It is completely atypical. It is pure and unrestrained creativity. This characteristic positions it at the heart of the enigma of being and of its genesis. Its exclusive properties are powerful and fecund. To a certain extent we can approach them with logic, through the new logic of ur-causality, which, as we know, is the metaphysics of all possible worlds. (I speak of this in two chapters of *La nouvelle physique de l'esprit*/The New Physics of the Spirit-Mind.)

Ur-causality is not of this world. Unlike partial endo-causality, it belongs to the world of transcendence. It appears as a kind of "creative principle," creator of the universe and of itself, because to be ur-causal means to enjoy absolute freedom. It means being and doing what one decides to be and do—without external restriction or constraint.

At present, here is how ur-causality—the creative principle par excellence—engenders the possibility of an ur-after. Here I quote myself once again:

> This "principle"—that we might be tempted to call god or divine and why not?—can maintain a privileged connection with the creatures of its creation. It can . . . if it decides to do so.
>
> This possible connection is no longer supral and immanent as before. It is ur-causal and transcendent. It has the ability to offer a true survival following death, perhaps for eternity, for its creatures. But what does the word "eternity" means in this context where the notion of time disappears? Because with ur-causality everything becomes possible. Everything is conceivable. All possible outcomes live in the "creative principle."[7]

The possible survival of what we might choose to call a "transcendent soul," or quite simply a "soul," defines the ur-after. It is a possibility but not a certainty. It is arbitrary and undecidable because it comes from an ur-causal decision that is intrinsically fluctuating and reversible. My quote continues:

> The ur-after is a transcendent hereafter, which pure ur-causality or endo-causality make perfectly conceivable. It is a gift. An unfathomable and mysterious gift whose existence is not demonstrable. . . . It is acquired through the "grace" of an ur-causal initiative.

Philosophy can speculate about it, but science will never be able to say the least thing about it. Each person is free to believe in it or to not believe in it.[8]

In short, the ur-after is an optional hereafter that can choose (or not) to create for each one of us, after the death of the body, the ur-causal "plan" or "principle" that will be at the origin of all that is. It is a "mystical hereafter."

The ur-after can only be apprehended by the understanding of the heart. By the way, Antoine de St. Exupéry stressed this in saying, "One sees clearly only with the heart." Krishnamurti confirmed that "deep seeing does not come through the brain." Enlightenment and self-transformation do not come through thought processes. This is the realm of the heart and of unconditional love.

In the end, if it is given to someone to survive in a hereafter, then that person becomes immortal. Or rather, they become "atemporal" because the notion of time, in this state, loses all relevance. It also then becomes conceivable that an ur-causal relatedness allows that person to maintain a privileged connection with those who are living. And to appear to them?

THE END OF THE ROAD . . .

In the final analysis, we discern two hereafters. This number, by the way, is not strictly limited since further speculation will bring perhaps other ways of thinking about survival and the hereafter. This calls to mind Georg Cantor (1845–1918), the mathematician of the infinite. His work (which was very poorly accepted by his peers) showed that there is an infinity of different infinities. Cantor called them "transfinite numbers." Before his revelations, we were familiar with two infinites only: a present infinite and a potential infinite. Cantor ushered in a new and fascinating chapter in the history of mathematics.

Whatever the ur-after might be, since it tosses us into dizzying reaches of transcendence, it remains a great unknown. In fact, a possible "ur-causal principle" or transcendent principle—shall we say, even, a divine principle, or God?—fundamentally decides what is up to it to decide.

No one can know its choices, no one can formulate the laws concerning it. Essentially, the ur-causal principle is unknowable and immeasurable. It is, in a word, undecidable. No one can put it in a box or in an equation.

Only humility allows it to be approached, in the modest limits of what is possible.

It can, however, choose to address itself to us since everything is permissible for it. Can it be that certain people manage to hear its messages? I am thinking of certain kinds of channeling. I am also thinking of Arlette Triolaire's meta-connection.[9] Clearly we have here only rigorously indemonstrable hypotheses. In this area where proof is doubtful or even nonexistent, the utmost caution is required. (See, however, the strange case of Padre Pio on page 126.)

In any event, we see, by following this somewhat abstract detour, that nothing allows us to assert that bodily death is the end of the road. With two hereafters being presented to us, bodily death might only be a movement through, a transition to other forms of existence or toward other planes of being. This idea, or rather this intuition, is not new. It has already been formulated many times.

Is death the ultimate end? This is an enormous question, which the towering poet Victor Hugo reformulated in this way: "Of what butterfly is this earthly life the caterpillar?"

If, for Immanuel Kant, death is the passing from time to eternity, it is perhaps also a window that opens on the absolute. Nothing allows us to see in death a pure and simple disappearance or the definitive negation of the incarnated being. As we have learned, the incarnated being extends outside its envelope of flesh through its double related-ness: through it supral relatedness and through its ur-causal relatedness. The first produces meta-consciousness; the second fades away into the ur-after. These two relatednesses are bridges toward an afterlife steeped in life: Isn't this perspective a wonderful source of hope and meaning?

It's interesting to note that there are stunning and verifiable facts which suggest, lacking any credible conventional explanation, that a transcendence—therefore an ur-causal dimension, I believe—would manifest here and there in our immanent world.

As proof of this I submit, subject to the results of a more rigorous study, of course, the following:

Do miracles exist? My answer is yes and is supported by proofs. For example, there is the case of Padre Pio. This Catholic priest, an Italian born in 1887 who died in 1968 and was canonized in 2002, was exhumed in 2008 and—surprise—his body, which had not undergone any special treatment, was in a state of perfect preservation. This violates all biochemical laws! . . . Other known cases of perfectly preserved bodies—which sometimes even exude a pleasant scent—exist in the world. Remarkably, in all such cases the body belonged to beings of high spiritual elevation. This was the case of the great Tibetan Buddhist monk Dudjom Rinpoche: his body remained unchanged in a posture of meditation.[10]

Such cases, of course, are extremely rare. I would like to add that the pleasant scent mentioned is precisely what we call "the scent of saintliness." This expression is to be taken quite literally!

In concluding, it's the right moment to recall that there are several ways of looking at facts and at things. As Saint Bonaventure said, we can regard them as objects or as signs. Facts, objects, or signs? Might these signs sometimes come forth from the ur-after? Let's not be too hasty in rejecting this possibility, even if it rocks our beliefs and roughs up our prejudices. Remember that this possibility harbors a treasure that shines with life.

It opens our hearts and our minds to a luminous and promising vista—that of the mysteries of the infinite.

EMMANUEL RANSFORD, epistemologist and physicist, is also a lecturer, author, and independent researcher. Dissatisfied by materialism and seeking a different model of reality, he has, through his work, explored the foundations of modern physics and, in particular, the strange behavior of quantum systems and how it may contribute to quantum consciousness. In France, his ideas have been summarized in Jean-Pierre Girard's *Encyclopédie du paranormal* (Encyclopedia of the Paranormal), for which he wrote the preface. Additionally, he has published numerous articles on his research and is the author of *La nouvelle physique de l'esprit* (The New Physics of the Spirit-Mind) and *Les racines physiques de l'esprit* (The Physical Underpinnings of the Spirit-Mind).

Notes

CHAPTER 1.
THE FIRST GOOD REASON

1. Gallup poll, 1993; *U.S. News & World Report,* 1997; Garlic and Smith, "Reports from the Beyond," 187–215.
2. Blanke et al., "Stimulating Illusory Own-body Perceptions," 269–70 and by the same authors, "Out-of-body Experience and Autoscopy of Neurological Origin," 243–58.
3. Morzelle, *Tout commence . . . après* (Everything Begins Afterward).
4. van Lommel et al., "Near-Death Experience in Survivors of Cardiac Arrest: A Prospective Study in the Netherlands."
5. Charbonier, *L'après-vie existe* (The Afterlife Exists), 70–73.
6. Blum, *La science devant la survie de l'âme* (Science Faces the Survival of the Soul), 42.
7. Morzelle, *Tout commence . . . après* (Everything Begins Afterward).
8. Blum, *La science devant la survie de l'âme* (Science Faces the Survival of the Soul), 67.
9. Ring and Cooper, "Near-death and Out-of-body Experiences in the Blind"; Ring, *Mindsight.*
10. van Lommel et al., "Near-Death Experience in Survivors of Cardiac Arrest."

11. Ibid.; see also the *Journal of Near-Death Studies*, vol. 25, no. 4 (2007), entirely devoted to this case.

CHAPTER 5.
THE FIFTH GOOD REASON

1. The details of this anecdote, which turned my life upside down, are written up in Charbonier, *Les preuves scientifiques d'une Vie après la vie* (Scientific Proof of a Life after This Life), 22–23.
2. Déthiollaz and Fourrier, *États modifiés de conscience* (Altered States of Consciousness), 212.
3. Charbonier, *La médecine face à l'au-delà* (Medicine Confronts the Hereafter), 17–30.

CHAPTER 7.
THE SEVENTH GOOD REASON

1. Prieur, *Les morts ont donné signe de vie* (The Dead Have Given Us Signs of Life).
2. Ragueneau, *L'autre côté de la vie* (The Other Side of Life).
3. Lerma, *Into the Light*.
4. Since 1993 the author has published numerous editions of this book (in French). See, for example, Brune, *Les morts nous parlent* (The Dead Speak to Us), vols. 1 and 2 (2009).
5. For more information (in French) see www.sourcedevietoulouse .com, www.infinitude.asso.fr, or www.christophebarbe.com (accessed November 18, 2014).
6. Charbonier, *Les preuves scientifiques d'une Vie après la vie* (Scientific Proof of a Life After This Life), 200–207.
7. Lines, *Quand l'au-delà se dévoile* (When the Hereafter Appears), 113.
8. Barbé, *Le langage de l'invisible* (The Language of the Invisible), 122–23.
9. Brune, *Les morts nous parlent* (The Dead Speak to Us), 28.

10. Ibid., 134–40.

11. Riotte, *Ces voix venues de l'au-delà* (Voices That Have Come from the Hereafter), 130.

CONCLUSION

1. See the details of this survey (in French) in Charbonier, "Enquête: Que sait on vraiment de la vie après la mort? (Survey: What we really know about life after death)" in the magazine *Ça m'intéresse*, April 2011, found on the author's website: http://jean-jacques.charbonier. fr/v2/uploads/gaelle/Ca%20minteresse1.gif.

APPENDIX. PSYCHOMATTER— FROM QUANTA TO THE HEREAFTER

1. A number of books provide citations of objective and statistical proof of telepathy. They include Dean Radin, *The Conscious Universe: The Scientific Proof of Psychic Phenomena* and Marcel Odier, *Phénomènes Insolites*. See also books by Rupert Sheldrake.

2. Ransford, *La nouvelle physique de l'esprit* (The New Physics of the Spirit-Mind), and *Les racines physiques de l'esprit* (The Physical Underpinnings of the Spirit-Mind).

3. Ransford, "Au-delà et physique quantique (The Hereafter and Quantum Physics)" and Triolaire, "Qu'est-ce qui se trame dans l'invisible? (What's Going on in the Invisible World)," from *Quantique et inconscient* (Quantum Mechanics and the Unconscious).

4. Ransford, "Paranormal et microphysique: Une approche par la psy-chomatière (Paranormal and Particle Physics: An Approach through Psychomatter)."

5. Girard, *La science et les phénomènes de l'au-delà* (Science and the Phenomena of the Hereafter).

6. Ransford, "La nouvelle physique, le transpersonnel et le divin en nous (The New Physics, the Transpersonal and the Divine in Us)."

7. Ransford, "Au-delà et physique quantique (Hereafter and Quantum Physics)."

8. Ibid.

9. Triolaire, *Quantique et inconscient* (Quantum Mechanics and the Unconscious).

10. This quotation is a mixture of sentences extracted from the article by Emmanuel Ransford, "Qu'est-ce que l'information quantique?" (What Is Quantum Information?) in *Sacrée Planète* (Blessed Planet), no. 43, Dec. 2010–Jan. 2011 and from his interview, "La psychomatière: Une nouvelle physique de l'esprit (Psychomatter: A New Physics of the Spirit-Mind)" in *Enquêtes de Santé* (Investigations on Health), no. 8, Aug.–Sept. 2011.

Bibliography

Barbé, Christophe. *Le langage de l'invisible* (The Language of the Invisible). Berlin: Kymzo, 2006.

———. *Comment les morts s'expriment* (How the Dead Communicate). Berlin: Kymzo, 2007.

———. *Signes de survivance* (Survival Signs). Berlin: Kymzo, 2009.

Baudouin, B. *Near-Death Experiences.* Milan: De Vecchi Publishing, 2006.

Beauregard, Mario, and D. O'Leary. *The Spiritual Brain: A Neuroscientist's Case for the Existence of the Soul.* New York: HarperOne, 2007.

Beauregard, Mario, Jean Jacques Charbonier, Sylvie Dethiollaz, J. P. Jourdan, E. S. Mercier, Raymond Moody, S. Parnia, P. van Eersel, and P. van Lommel. *Actes du colloque de Martigues du 17 juin 2006: Premières rencontres internationales sur l'Expérience de Mort Imminente* (Proceedings of the Congress at Martigues, June 17, 2006: First International Meetings on Near-Death Experiences). Lyon, France: S17 Production, 2007.

Benhedi, L., and J. Morisson. *Les NDE: Expériences de mort imminente* (NDEs: Experiences of Provisional Death). Paris: Editions Dervy, 2008.

Bessière, Richard. *Les morts parlent aux vivants* (The Dead Speak to the Living). Paris: Trajectoire, 2005.

Blanke, O., S. Ortigue, T. Landis, and M. Seeck. "Stimulating Illusory Own-body Perceptions." *Nature* 419 (2002): 269–70.

Blanke, O., T. Landis, L. Spinelli, and M. Seeck. "Out-of-body Experience and Autoscopy of Neurological Origin." *Brain* 127 (2004): 243–58.

Blanc-Garin, Jacques, and Monique Blanc-Garin. *En communion avec nos défunts: Dans l'infinitude de l'amour* (Communing with Our Dead: In the Infinity of Love). Monaco: Alphée/Editions du Rocher, 2007.

———. *L'infinitude de la vie: Communication avec les défunts, recherches et preuves* (Life's Infinity: Communication with the Dead, Research and Proof). Monaco: Alphée/Editions du Rocher, 2009.

Blum, Jean. *La science devant la survie de l'âme: NDE expérience* (Science Faces the Survival of the Soul: The NDE Experience). Monaco: Alphée/Editions du Rocher, 2010.

Bouvier, Hélène. *Mission des âmes dans l'au-delà* (The Soul's Mission in the Hereafter). Paris: Edition Le Temps Présent, 2009.

Brune, François. *Les morts nous parlent* (The Dead Speak to Us). Paris: Philippe Lebaud, 2002.

———. *Les morts nous parlent* (The Dead Speak to Us), new edition, vol. 2. Escalquens, France: Editions Oxus, 2006.

———. *Les morts nous parlent* (The Dead Speak to Us), vols. 1 and 2. Paris: Le Livre de Poche, 2009.

———. *Les morts nous aiment* (The Dead Love Us). Paris: Editions Le Temps Présent, 2009.

Canivenq, Nicole. *L'arbre du choix* (The Tree of Choice). Paris: Editions Le Temps Présent, 2010.

Chambon, Olivier. *La medicine psychédélique* (Psychedelic Medicine). Paris: Les Arènes, 2009.

Chambon, Olivier, and Laurent Huguelit. *Le chamane et le psy* (The Shaman and the Shrink). Paris: Mama Editions, 2011.

Charbonier, Jean Jacques. *L'après-vie existe* (The Afterlife Exists). Montélimar, France: CLC Editions, 2006.

———. *La mort décodée* (Death Deciphered). Paris: Guy Trédaniel, 2008.

————. *Les preuves scientifiques d'une Vie après la vie* (Scientific Proof of a Life after This Life). Paris: Editions Exergue, 2008.

————. *La médecine face à l'au-delà* (Medicine Confronts the Hereafter). Paris: Guy Trédaniel, 2010.

Chateigner, Karine. *Le nouveau livre des esprits* (The New Book about Spirits). Paris: Cercle Spirite Allan Kardec, 2002.

Chopra, Deepak. *Life after Death.* New York: Harmony Books, 2006.

Coulombe, Marylène. *Les morts nous donnent signe de vie* (The Dead Give Us Signs of Life). Sonchamp, France: Edimag, 2005.

Dalai Lama. *Sleeping, Dreaming, and Dying.* Somerville, Mass.: Wisdom Publications, 1997.

————. *Voyage aux confins de l'esprit.* Paris: J'ai lu, 2010.

Decker, Michèle. *La vie de l'autre côté* (Life on the Other Side). Paris: J'ai lu, 2005.

Descamps, Marc Alain. *Les expériences de mort imminente et l'après-vie* (Near-Death Experiences and the Afterlife). Labege, France: Editions Dangles, 2008.

Déthiollaz, Sylvie, and Claude Charles Fourrier. *États modifiés de conscience: NDE, OBE, et autres expériences aux frontières de l'esprit* (Altered States of Consciousness: NDE, OBE, and Other Experiences on the Outer Reaches of the Mind). Lausanne, France: Favre, 2011.

Dray, Maryvonne, and Yvon Dray. *Karine après la vie* (Karine after Her Life). Paris: Albin Michel, 2002.

Dron, Nicole. *45 secondes d'éternité: Mes souvenirs de l'au-delà* (45 Seconds of Eternity: My Memories of the Hereafter). Berlin: Kymzo, 2009.

Eadie, Betty J. *Dans les bras de la lumière* (Cradled by the Light). Paris: Pocket, 2006.

Eccles, John C. *How the Self Controls Its Brain.* Paris: Springer-Verlag, 1994.

Elsaesser Valarino, Evelyn. *Le pays d'Ange* (The Country of Angels). Toulon, France: Les Presses du Midi, 2008.

Fontaine, Janine. *La médecine des trois corps* (Medicine for the Three Bodies). Paris: J'ai lu, 2005.

Garlic, H., and Ina Smith, eds. "Reports from the Beyond: A Qualitative Study on Near-death Experiences in Germany." In *Near-Death*. Constance, Germany: UVK, 1999.

Girard, Jean-Pierre. *Encyclopédie du paranormal* (Encyclopedia of the Paranormal). Paris: Trajectoire, 2005.

———. *Encyclopédie de l'au-delà* (Encyclopedia of the Hereafter). Paris: Trajectoire, 2006.

———. *La science et les phénomènes de l'au-delà* (Science and Phenomena of the Hereafter). Monaco: Alphée/Editions du Rocher, 2010.

Greyson, Bruce. "Incidence and Correlates of Near-death Experiences in a Cardiac Care Unit." *General Hospital Psychiatry* 25 (2003): 269–76.

Grof, Stanislav. *The Cosmic Game.* Albany, N.Y.: SUNY Press, 1998.

———. *The Ultimate Journey: Consciousness and the Mystery of Death.* Santa Cruz, Calif.: MAPS, 2006.

Kardec, Allan. *The Book on Mediums.* Newburyport, Mass.: Weiser Books, 1970.

———. *The Spirits' Book.* New York: Cosimo Classics, 2005.

Kübler-Ross, Elisabeth. *The Tunnel and the Light.* Boston: Da Capo Press, 1999.

———. *On Death and Dying.* New York: Routledge, 2009.

Lannaud, Patrick. *Témoignages et preuves de survie* (Survival Accounts and Verifications). Paris: Editions Le Temps Présent, 2008.

La Revue De L'Au-Delà (The Magazine of the Hereafter). Paris: Menssana, 1997.

Laszlo, Ervin. *Science and the Akashic Field.* Rochester, Vt.: Inner Traditions, 2007.

Le Gall, Jean Marie. *Contacts avec l'au-delà* (Contacts with the Hereafter). Paris: Editions Fernand Lanore, 2006.

Le Magazine De L'INREES (The INREES Journal), INREES: Institut de recherche sur les expériences extraordinaires (Research Institute on Extraordinary Experiences), Paris.

Lerma, John. *Into the Light*. Pompton Plains, N.J.: New Page Books, 2007.

Leshan, Lawrence. *The Medium, the Mystic, and the Physicist: Toward a Theory of the Paranormal*. New York: Helios Press, 2003.

Lines, Yves. *Quand l'au-delà se dévoile* (When the Hereafter Appears). Hescamps, France: JMG Editions, 2006.

McTaggart, Lynne. *The Intention Experiment: Using Your Thoughts to Change Your Life and the World*. New York: Free Press, 2007.

Martin, J. *Des signes par milliers* (Signs by the Thousands). Paris: Editions Le Temps Présent, 2011.

Maurer, D. *Les expériences de mort imminente* (Near-Death Experiences). Monaco: Editions du Rocher, 2005.

Monde du graal (The World of the Grail) magazine. Montreuil-sous-Bois, France: Éditions du Graal, n.d.

Moody, Raymond. *The Last Laugh*. Newburyport, Mass.: Hampton Roads Publishing, 1999.

———. *Life after Life*. New York: Harper, 2001.

———. *Glimpses of Eternity: Sharing a Loved One's Passage from this Life to the Next*. New York: Guideposts, 2010.

Morse, Melvin. *Closer to the Light: Learning from Children's Near-Death Experiences*. New York: Villard Books, 1990.

———. *La Divine Connexion* (The Divine Connection). Paris: Le Jardin des Livres, 2002.

———. *Le Contact Divin* (The Divine Contact). Paris: Le Jardin des Livres, 2005.

Moulin, Anne Marie. *Le papillon libéré* (The Butterfly Set Free). Paris: Editions Le Temps Présent, 2009.

Morzelle, J. *Tout commence . . . après: Mes rencontres avec l'au-delà* (Everything Begins . . . Afterward: My Encounters with the Hereafter). N.p.: CLC Editions, 2007.

Murakami, K. *The Divine Code of Life*. Hillsboro, Ore.: Beyond Words Publishing, 2006.

NDE Magazine, Le magazine de l'au-delà et de la vie après la mort (NDE

Magazine: The Magazine of the Hereafter and of Life after Death). Nice, France, n.d.

Odier, Marcel. *Phénomènes Insolites*. Lausanne, France: Favre, 2007.

Parasciences. Hescamps, France: JMG Editions, n.d.

Parnia, S., D. G. Waller, R. Yeates, and P. Fenwick. "A Qualitative and Quantitative Study of the Incidence, Features and Aetiology of Near-Death Experiences in Cardiac Arrest Survivors." *Resuscitations* 48 (2001): 149–56.

Prieur, Jean. *Les morts ont donné signes de vie* (The Dead Have Given Us Signs of Life). Paris: Editions Fernand Lanore, 1990.

Radin, Dean. *The Conscious Universe: The Scientific Proof of Psychic Phenomena*. New York: Harper, 1997.

Ragueneau, Philippe. *L'autre côté de la vie* (The Other Side of Life). Monaco: Editions du Rocher, 1997.

Ransford, Emmanuel. "Paranormal et microphysique: Une approche par la psychomatière (Paranormal and Particle Physics: An Approach through Psychomatter)." In Jean-Pierre Girard, *Encyclopédie du paranormal* (Encyclopedia of the Paranormal). Paris: Trajectoire, 2005.

———. "La nouvelle physique, le transpersonnel et le divin en nous (The New Physics, the Transpersonal and the Divine in the US)." *3ᵉ Millénaire* (3rd Millennium) 85, 2007.

———. *La nouvelle physique de l'esprit: Pour une nouvelle science de la matière* (The New Physics of the Spirit-Mind: Toward a New Science of Matter). Paris: Editions Le Temps Présent, 2007.

———. *Les racines physiques de l'esprit* (The Physical Underpinnings of the Spirit-Mind). Aubagne Cedex, France: Editions Quintessence, 2009.

———. "Au-delà et physique quantique (The Hereafter and Quantum Physics)." In Jean-Pierre Girard, *La science et les phénomènes de l'au-delà* (Science and Phenomena of the Hereafter). Monaco: Alphée/Editions du Rocher, 2010.

Rauzy, D. *L'éveil des nouveaux chamans: Une approche holistique de la vie* (New Shamans Awaken). Paris: Guy Trédaniel, 2008.

Rawlings, Maurice. *Beyond Death's Door*. New York: Bantam, 1991.

Ring, Kenneth. *Life at Death: A Scientific Investigation of the Near-Death Experience*. N.p.: Coward, McCann & Geoghegan, 1980.

———. *Sur la frontière de la vie*. Paris: Éditions Robert Laffont, 1982. (See also a later edition of *Sur la frontière de la vie* translated by Muriel American Lesterlin with a preface by Raymond Moody. Monaco: Alphée/Editions du Rocher, 2008.)

———. *Mindsight: Near-Death and Out-of-Body Experiences in the Blind*. Palo Alto, Calif.: William James Center for Consciousness Studies, 2009.

Ring, Kenneth, and Sharon Cooper. "Near-death and Out-of-body Experiences in the Blind: A Study of Apparent Eyeless Vision." *Journal of Near-Death Studies* 16, no. 2 (1997): 101–47.

Riotte, Jean. *Ces voix venues de l'au-delà* (Voices That Have Come from the Hereafter). Paris: France Loisirs, 2003.

Sabom, M. *Light and Death: One Doctor's Fascinating Account of Near-Death Experiences*. New York: Zondervan, 1998.

Sheldrake, Rupert. *Seven Experiments That Could Change the World*. Rochester, Vt.: Park Street Press, 2002.

Sogyal Rinpoche. *The Tibetan Book of Living and Dying*. New York: Harper, 1992.

Thigou, Sergui. *La violence faite à l'esprit* (Doing Violence to the Mind). Paris: Qetzal Podi, 2002.

Triolaire, Arlette. *Quantique et inconscient* (Quantum Mechanics and the Unconscious). Paris: Editions Le Temps Présent, 2011.

Van Eersel, Patrice. *La source noire: révélations aux portes de la mort* (The Black Spring: Revelations from the Gates of Death). Paris: Le Livre de Poche, 1987.

Van Cauwelaert, Didier. *Un aller simple*. Paris: Le Livre de Poche, 1995.

———. *La vie interdite* (The Forbidden Life). Paris: Le Livre de Poche, 1999.

———. *One-Way*. New York: Other Press, 2003.

————. *La maison des lumières* (The House of Light). Paris: Le Livre de Poche, 2011.

van Lommel, Pim. *Consciousness Beyond Life*. New York: HarperOne, 2010.

van Lommel, Pim, R. Van Wees, V. Meyers, and I. Elferich. "Near-Death Experience in Survivors of Cardiac Arrest: A Prospective Study in the Netherlands." *The Lancet* 358 (2001): 2039–45.

Vermeulen, Danielle. *NDE et expériences mystiques d'hier et d'aujourd'hui* (NDEs and Mystical Experiences from the Past and from Today). Paris: Editions Le Temps Présent, 2007.

Vignaud, Henry. *En contact avec l'invisible* (In Contact with the Invisible). Paris: InterÉditions, 2011.

Wickland, Carl A. *Thirty Years among the Dead*. N.p.: Mokelumne Hill Press, 1996.

Zeidler, Nadine (channeling Vladik). *Tu seras ma voix: Messages de Vladik à sa mere* (You Will Be My Voice: Messages from Vladik to His Mother). Quebec: Louise Courteau, 2010.

Index